THE COMPLETE GUIDE
TO LOWERING
YOUR CHOLESTEROL

Books in the Healthy Home Library Series from St. Martin's Paperbacks

A Woman's Guide to Vitamins, Herbs and Supplements
by Deborah Mitchell

The Complete Book of Nutritional Healing
by Deborah Mitchell

The Complete Guide to Living Well with Diabetes
by Winifred Conkling

The Concise Encyclopedia of Women's Sexual and Reproductive Health
by Deborah Mitchell

25 Medical Tests Your Doctor Should Tell You About . . .
by Deborah Mitchell

52 Foods and Supplements for a Healthy Heart
by Deborah Mitchell

How to Live Well With Early Alzheimer's
by Deborah Mitchell

The Anti-Cancer Food and Supplement Guide
by Debora Yost

The Family Guide to Vitamins, Herbs, and Supplements
by Deborah Mitchell

The Complete Guide to Lowering Your Cholesterol
by Mary Mihaly

THE COMPLETE GUIDE TO LOWERING YOUR CHOLESTEROL

Your All-in-One Resource for a Heart-Healthy Life

Mary Mihaly

A Lynn Sonberg Book

St. Martin's Paperbacks

Notice: This book is intended as a reference volume only, not as a medical manual. The information given here is designed to help you make informed decisions about your health. It is not intended as a substitute for any treatment that may have been prescribed by your doctor. If you suspect that you have a medical problem, we urge you to seek competent medical help.

Mention of specific companies, organizations, or authorities in this book does not imply endorsement by the author or publisher, nor does mention of specific companies, organizations, or authorities imply that they endorse this book, its author or the publisher.

Internet addresses given in this book were accurate at the time it went to press.

THE COMPLETE GUIDE TO LOWERING YOUR CHOLESTEROL

Copyright © 2011 by Lynn Sonberg Book Associates.

All rights reserved.

For information address St. Martin's Press, 175 Fifth Avenue, New York, NY 10010.

EAN: 978-0-312-53419-6

Printed in the United States of America

St. Martin's Paperbacks edition / February 2011

St. Martin's Paperbacks are published by St. Martin's Press, 175 Fifth Avenue, New York, NY 10010.

10 9 8 7 6 5 4 3 2 1

O 1021 0258189 3

CONTENTS

THE COMPLETE GUIDE TO LOWERING YOUR CHOLESTEROL

PART I

Cholesterol and Heart Disease:
What You Need to Know

CHAPTER ONE

Understanding Cholesterol, the New Epidemic

Does it seem as if half the people you know are taking medication to lower their cholesterol levels? If so, your impression is on target: More than 36 million Americans, as many as 18 percent of some ethnic groups, have been diagnosed with "high risk" cholesterol—the danger zone for heart disease. When the measure is for "borderline high risk," those numbers triple to more than 100 million Americans who need to treat their unhealthy cholesterol levels. With numbers like that, just about everyone who is at all health-conscious has thought about their cholesterol. We worry about cholesterol because, when our levels are too high, our risk of developing heart disease also increases. And when our high cholesterol is accompanied by other heart-risk factors, such as diabetes and high blood pressure, the threat of heart disease grows even more.

If you or someone in your family has been told their cholesterol levels are too high, you might be feeling uncertain, or even a little frightened, about your future. After all, we've all known someone who fell victim to heart disease. In fact it is the leading cause of death for men *and* women in the U.S.

If you are a woman, you may think you're immune to serious heart disease, but here is the reality: Heart disease kills one in every 2.6 women in America. About 37 percent of women in this country will die of cardiovascular disease

(CVD), including coronary heart disease (CHD), stroke and other heart diseases. The rate is substantially higher in women of color. Yet, a study by the American Heart Association (AHA) found that only 13 percent of American women believe that heart disease and stroke are their greatest health risk.

Here's the good news: Many people can lower their cholesterol levels, and avoid the specter of heart disease, by switching to a heart-healthy lifestyle. The cornerstones of such a plan are exercise and good nutrition. Many people also choose to include one or more thoughtfully selected nutritional supplements in their new lifestyle.

But where to begin? That's where this book comes in. We will introduce you to a range of choices that can enhance your health, lower your cholesterol levels and help you avoid heart disease. You may even be able to reach those goals naturally, as many have, without the aid of prescription drugs; others adopt their new heart-healthy choices while taking prescribed medications, and some find that their cholesterol levels drop so much they can stop taking those drugs forever.

IT'S ALL ABOUT CHOICES

Everyone's system is different. What *The Complete Guide to Lowering Your Cholesterol* offers you is a range of choices to discuss with your doctor and, if you choose, adopt those that you think can help lower your cholesterol. This is a guidebook; use it to make a plan for building your heart health.

The core of your plan will be a specific diet, exercise and supplementation practice. You will learn which foods and nutrients help prevent cardiovascular disease, and you will be given guidelines for designing your own healthy eating plan.

The Complete Guide to Lowering Your Cholesterol doesn't stop with those basics; it goes on to show you easy meal planning, shopping and organizing strategies so that you can prepare heart-healthy meals every day. We will walk through your real life, too. We all eat in restaurants, at family feasts and at tailgate parties, and you will learn to make smart, satisfying choices in those tempting situations as well.

YOU'VE GOT TO HAVE HEART

It's the organ that never takes a break: Your heart beats about 100,000 times a day, pumping blood—with its life-giving oxygen and nutrients—throughout your body. In seventy-five years, this tireless organ beats more than 2.7 billion times. No wonder we need to take care of it!

You learned about the heart and how it works in grade school, but here's a quick refresher course. Located near the center of your chest, your heart is made of four chambers. The upper chambers, called the left and right atrium, are smaller than those below—the left and right ventricle.

Your blood follows a prescribed path through your heart: Veins carry "used" blood, low in oxygen, to the right atrium. From there, it flows into the right ventricle and exits via the pulmonary (a word that means "relating to the lungs") artery. Next stop is the lungs themselves, where the blood is infused with oxygen and carbon dioxide is removed.

From the lungs, the newly oxygenated blood enters the pulmonary veins and travels to the left ventricle. This chamber is the real powerhouse of the heart; here your "clean" blood is given a giant push out into the aorta, into your major arteries and on to the various parts of your body.

It is the coronary arteries that bring blood and oxygen to the heart. When one of them becomes obstructed (with cholesterol buildup or "plaque," for instance), and the heart muscle can't get enough oxygen, the part of the heart that's connected to that artery will die within about thirty minutes. That's how a heart attack happens; perhaps because the left ventricle works so hard, it is the chamber most vulnerable to heart attacks.

WHAT, EXACTLY, IS CHOLESTEROL?

Measuring cholesterol is a simple matter; it's done with a blood test in your doctor's office. The levels are standardized throughout the medical profession, and you'll read about those numbers, and what they mean, in Chapter 2. That's where you will learn the difference between HDL, the "good cholesterol," and LDL, the "bad cholesterol," and how both levels affect your heart health.

But what, exactly, are those tests measuring? What is cholesterol?

Almost every expert describes cholesterol with the same terms: It's a waxy, fatty substance. I think of it as lard that sticks to the insides of your arteries and eventually hardens into plaque. If your mother made pie crusts years ago, she probably used a vegetable shortening that resembles lard. For those too young to recall pie crusts that didn't come prepackaged, just visualize white-ish peanut butter. That's what cholesterol is like.

TOO MUCH OF A NECESSARY THING

That sticky, waxy material called cholesterol plays a needed role in your body. It is manufactured in your liver and can be found inside all of our cells. Cholesterol helps to manufacture adrenal hormones and vitamin D, the "sunshine vitamin" that you'll learn much more about in Chapter 7, where we discuss food supplements and vitamins. It helps to produce bile and sex hormones, and builds and maintains the outer layers (membranes) of cells. Cholesterol is so necessary to our well-being, in fact, that manufacturers even add it to baby formula because infants need it for normal development.

Cholesterol also is needed to form brain cells and transmit nerve impulses across the brain, and it helps you to digest food—but a little bit goes a long way.

You also absorb cholesterol from the foods you eat. When you eat foods high in saturated fat and trans fats, are overweight or have a family history of high cholesterol levels, you absorb more, and it begins to stick to the insides of your artery walls. Bit by bit, over time, it builds up and hardens. When that happens, it's called "plaque," much like the plaque that can build up on your teeth. Eventually it can lead to *atherosclerosis*, or hardening of the arteries.

Most often, when you hear someone talking about heart disease, he or she is referring to atherosclerosis. Sometimes it's called "coronary artery disease." High cholesterol levels are one of the top risk factors for all heart disease; studies show that the higher your cholesterol, the higher your chances of developing heart disease—the top killer of men and women in the U.S.—and having a heart attack. And more than 1.2 million adults in this country have heart attacks every year.

You will read much more about fats and healthy eating strategies in Chapter 4, "You Are What You Eat," and Chapter 5, "Your TLC Eating Plan." For this discussion, just keep in mind that meats, eggs and dairy products are especially high in saturated fat, and hydrogenated vegetable oils are the most common source of trans fats. (We won't recommend that you cut saturated fats out of your diet entirely; in fact, new studies show that saturated fats can be beneficial, especially compared to the high-glycemic carbs some people eat to replace the fats—but we're getting ahead of ourselves here.)

High cholesterol is one of those tricky conditions that doesn't exhibit symptoms. It's diagnosed with simple blood tests that give you specific measures of your cholesterol levels. You'll learn more about those tests, who should take them, what they measure and how to know if your cholesterol levels are too high, in Chapter 2.

But even though it gives off no symptoms, high cholesterol does bring effects—and they're not good. One recent study of 19,000 men published in the *British Medical Journal* found that men in their middle years who smoke and have high blood pressure and high cholesterol will live an average of ten to fifteen years less than healthier men their age.

MUMMY HAD ATHEROSCLEROSIS, TOO

It turns out hardening of the arteries isn't a modern disease. CT scans of mummified bodies of Egyptians who lived 3,500 years ago found atherosclerosis in those who lived a more affluent lifestyle.

Published in *Journal of the American Medical Association* (JAMA), the study is a collaboration between scientists at four universities. Of twenty mummies in the Museum of Egyptian Antiquities in Cairo that were studied, sixteen were found with plaque in their arteries. Half of them were older than forty-five when they died; one was the body of Lady Rai, Queen Ahmose-Nefertari's nursemaid, who lived about three hundred years before Moses and died in about 1530 B.C. Most were in the court of the Pharaoh, who commonly ate meat from cattle, ducks and geese.

GOOD CHOLESTEROL, BAD CHOLESTEROL

When we measure cholesterol levels, we're actually measuring lipoproteins—the molecules that carry cholesterol in the blood. (Most people are surprised to learn that "high cholesterol" really refers to the molecules that carry it, rather than the cholesterol itself.) A lipoprotein is a molecule that contains both lipid (fat) and protein, and there are three main types.

- *LDL, or low-density lipoproteins.* These small, dense molecules carry cholesterol from your liver to your cells, and are known as the "bad" cholesterol. (You can remember it by telling yourself "L" stands for "lousy.") When it carries too much cholesterol for the cells to use, it deposits the cholesterol on the arterial walls—thus clogging the arteries, developing plaque and leading to heart disease.

- *HDL, or high-density lipoproteins.* HDL ("H" stands for "happy") carries cholesterol *away from* the arteries, actually helping to prevent plaque buildup and clogged arteries—and, consequently, heart disease—and deposits the cholesterol in the liver, where it's either broken down or expelled from the body. If you are lean, don't smoke cigarettes and exercise most days, chances are you have a high, healthy HDL level. Also, estrogen tends to boost HDL cholesterol levels, so women before menopause typically show higher HDL counts than men.

- *Triglycerides.* Found in blood plasma, triglycerides are fatty acids that combine with cholesterol to form plasma lipids, or blood fat. When you eat more calories than you use, the extra calories are converted into triglycerides and sent to fat cells for storage. You need some triglycerides stored in your body; you use them for energy when food isn't available, a process controlled by hormones. But eat more calories than you will eventually use, and the triglycerides remain in the form of stored fat.

As you read this book, keep in mind, too, that food isn't the only lifestyle factor that can raise your cholesterol to an unhealthy level. Other choices such as inactivity and smoking also contribute to high cholesterol. In a small portion of cases, certain medical conditions also can cause high levels.

The damage begins with injury to the thin lining, called an *endothelium*, inside your artery. This damage can be caused by any one of a number of conditions, including cigarette smoking, high blood pressure, diabetes or *hypercholesterolemia*—the cholesterol buildup itself. As LDL, or bad cholesterol, sweeps past the damaged spot, it enters the artery wall and stays there. Plaque eventually forms, and little by little, the space inside the artery narrows. Blood may try to heal the damaged spot, too, and form a clot, further clogging the artery.

By middle age or older, the narrowing has become severe and blood cannot get through the artery any more, causing pain. Plaques can rupture, calling on blood to clot inside the artery. If that happens in the brain, the result is a stroke; if it happens in the heart, it means a heart attack.

HOW TO PREVENT ATHEROSCLEROSIS

Although it progresses over years, atherosclerosis is absolutely preventable. That's why this book is being published! The American Heart Association cites three heart disease risk factors—aging, being male and heredity, including race—that we can do nothing about. However, they also list nine other risk factors that absolutely can be changed, treated or controlled by changing your lifestyle or taking medication.

- Tobacco smoke;
- High blood cholesterol;
- High blood pressure;
- Physical inactivity;
- Obesity and overweight;
- Diabetes mellitus;
- Stress;
- Alcohol; and
- Diet and nutrition.

WHO GETS HIGH CHOLESTEROL?

Would you believe, more people than not?

Autopsies done on soldiers killed in the Korean and Vietnam Wars revealed that up to three-quarters of them had beginning plaque formations in their arteries—and this was during the days of "the draft," when young men were drafted into the armed forces soon after their eighteenth birthdays!

Atherosclerosis is not an old man's disease—or an old woman's. Those soldiers' autopsies showed early atherosclerosis in 17 percent of soldiers who still were teenagers when they died.

Today, we know that a healthy forty-year-old has a 50 percent chance of developing serious atherosclerosis in his or her older years; most people older than sixty have some artery disease but may not notice any symptoms. And while men develop heart disease earlier than women (again, in large part because their systems are not protected by estrogen), women catch up to men in their later years, when both sexes are equally susceptible to heart disease.

CAN YOU BLAME IT ON MOM AND DAD?

Although most high cholesterol is caused by lifestyle choices and is preventable, the fact is there are several genetic disorders that do cause severely high blood cholesterol levels. They include:

- *Familial hypercholesterolemia.* This disorder is the most common form of inherited high cholesterol, striking about one person in every five hundred. People with familial hypercholesterolemia have high cholesterol levels and are at high risk of developing coronary artery disease. Tracking family history, taking the usual blood tests that measure cholesterol levels, and a stress test all will determine whether you have inherited it. The good news: Familial hypercholesterolemia can be treated with statin medications and lifestyle changes.

- *Familial combined hyperlipidemia.* People with FCH have large amounts of fat levels, including cholesterol, in their blood, causing both high cholesterol and high triglycerides. About 20 percent of Americans under age sixty who suffer from coronary artery disease also have FCH. It's a common cause of heart attacks in young people; treatment often involves a combination of lifestyle changes, statin meds and bile acid sequestrants—drugs that remove cholesterol from the body.

Collectively, genetic disorders cause fewer than 5 percent of all high cholesterol cases. Because their high cholesterol wasn't caused by lifestyle choices, people with these diseases need more aggressive treatments than lifestyle changes alone—though a diet that restricts fat and cholesterol, along with exercise, is always recommended.

Often, their treatment plans also will include higher-than-usual doses of medications in order to manage their cholesterol levels. These conditions cannot be taken lightly; many people diagnosed with both FH and FCH do, in fact, experience a heart attack in spite of careful management. Still, if the patient commits to a heart-healthy lifestyle and the right medication, he or she can thrive for years.

Aside from these inherited cholesterol disorders, genetics does play a role in many cases of high cholesterol levels—possibly the biggest role, some experts believe, even when a healthier lifestyle of exercise and better eating can remedy the problem.

That's because, regardless of your cholesterol levels, you depend on your level to remove excess cholesterol from your body. It's one of the liver's most important functions, and genetics, in large part, determines how well your liver performs. If your liver is just slightly underfunctioning, then a healthier lifestyle can boost its performance and reduce your cholesterol levels by 10 percent or more.

MOVING TOWARD A SOLUTION

If you or someone in your family has high cholesterol levels, then you're looking for a way to resolve the problem and get healthy again. That's where this book comes in: It is a reference to help you understand cholesterol and how to manage it.

You will read, in fact, about all of your options in lowering your cholesterol levels and reaching heart-healthy wellness in this book. For many of you, that wellness will come as a result of changing your life with healthier eating, dietary supplements, exercise and stress management. For others, cholesterol management will come by way of a more traditional route that includes medications. Or you may start with one plan and alter it—with your doctor's blessing—as you progress toward better health. Good health is a journey, not a destination, and you will always be working on that process.

For any physical condition, including high cholesterol, many of us find ourselves asking, "Conventional medicine, or alternative? Or some combination?" When that question occurs to you, your doctor's office should be your first stop. If your cholesterol levels are dangerously high, you may need a prescription to lower them quickly. If they are only slightly elevated, on the other hand, you may choose to follow the National Heart, Lung, and Blood Institute of the National Institutes of Health's "TLC Program" for lowering cholesterol levels—a regimen of food, supplements and exercise that will help you manage your cholesterol in a healthy way.

Or, you may be searching for an integrative plan—one that includes both a healthier lifestyle and prescription medicines.

So, you have some decisions to make, and this book will walk you through them. If you prefer an alternative, nonprescription treatment for your cholesterol, we will do our best to present the pros and cons of each food plan, exercise routine, nutritional supplement or stress-reducing technique, so you can be fully informed and prepared when you talk about your choices with your doctor. That's the core of this book, a presentation of natural, nonprescription choices for lowering cholesterol.

We've also provided basic information about statin (cholesterol-lowering) medications, those prescription drugs that lower cholesterol levels by limiting the amount of cholesterol produced in the liver.

We've tracked down the latest, most useful findings for reducing cholesterol, and you will find them all in *The Complete Guide to Lowering Your Cholesterol*.

CHAPTER TWO

What the Numbers Mean—Are You at Risk?

At some point, you will need to get your cholesterol tested—
and by "you," we mean every adult and teenager. So in this
chapter, I'm going to tell you everything you need to know
about this process . . . when to do it and what the numbers
mean. We'll also talk about heart disease risks—who is at
risk, what puts you there and what you can do about it. The
good news is, regardless of whether you are at high, medium
or low risk, you have plenty of choices for creating a healthier, more energetic, more productive future.

IT'S NOT JUST A TEST FOR THE OVER-FORTY
CROWD ANYMORE

Researchers are finding early signs of atherosclerosis in teenagers and young adults. In fact, a 2010 study by the Centers
for Disease Control found that one in five American teenagers is at risk for developing heart disease later in life, presenting either low levels of HDL (high-density lipoprotein,
the "good" cholesterol, you will remember), high LDL (low-
density lipoprotein) or high triglycerides. Most teens with
high cholesterol have at least one parent with the same problem, so heredity is sometimes a factor. Just as often, though,
high levels in kids are linked to a high-fat diet, obesity and
too little exercise.

Catching high cholesterol at an early age is a good thing; if the screening produces a low HDL (the "good" cholesterol, remember) or high LDL or triglycerides score in a young person, then he or she can pinpoint the behaviors that helped create the high cholesterol levels and incorporate healthier habits into their routines.

Even if your son or daughter is healthy, experts now recommend that everyone undergo cholesterol screening by age twenty and be tested again every five years.

Actually, calling it a "cholesterol screening" makes the test sound much more elaborate than it really is. In spite of its even more high-tech medical name, a "lipoprotein profile" or "lipid panel" is nothing more than a quick-and-easy blood test—the same test, whether you are eighteen years old or sixty-eight—but your life could depend on it. In this chapter, we will explore the testing procedure, and what the results of that test mean for you. We'll discuss additional tests and risk factors in Chapter 3.

TAKING A CHOLESTEROL TEST

Why do I need the test—what will it tell my doctor?

The standard test for checking your blood cholesterol levels is called a *lipid panel*. It will show your doctor a precise reading of your HDL, LDL and triglyceride levels. Ask your primary care physician to incorporate the test into your routine of regular visits; for many doctors, a cholesterol test is standard procedure. You might want a copy of the results for your own files, so you can track your progress over time.

Where should I take the test?

Usually your doctor will take your blood sample in his or her office. You might also see cholesterol tests offered at health expos and drugstores, and they require no preparation on your part except twelve hours of fasting—easy to accomplish;

just eat an early supper and have your blood tested the next morning before you eat breakfast. If you do have your cholesterol checked at a public screening, be sure to get the results in writing and share them with your physician.

The advantage to having your doctor do the test, however, is that your personal physician can assess more than the bottom-line numbers. Because the doctor knows you, he or she can analyze the test results in light of your family history, medical history, blood pressure and lifestyle factors.

How do I prepare for the test?

For the truest picture of your cholesterol profile, drink nothing but water for twelve hours before your test, and no alcohol for three days. Even during a scheduled office visit, the accuracy of a lipid panel can be thrown off if you had coffee or tea that morning, or drank alcohol during the past several days.

SCREENING KIDS FOR CHOLESTEROL

Fortunately, the American Academy of Pediatrics took the guesswork out of deciding whether your school-age child should undergo a cholesterol test. In July 2008, they recommended that children with a family history of high cholesterol levels or triglycerides, or a family history of early heart disease, should be screened. They define "family history of premature heart disease" as seeing the disease in male relatives fifty-five or younger, or female relatives sixty-five or younger.

They also advise cholesterol screening for overweight children (at or above the 85th percentile) and those who present other risk factors such as high blood pressure, smoking or diabetes.

Kids with any of these risk factors should be tested after age two and no later than age ten; if the fasting lipid profile shows results in the normal range, the test should be repeated in three to five years.

If your child is overweight or obese and the result shows high triglycerides or low HDL levels, the first recommendation will be to get the child's weight in the healthy range through exercise and sound nutrition. If your child is older than eight years and shows very high cholesterol levels (or high levels with a family history of early heart disease), your doctor might consider managing the child's cholesterol with medication, as well as lifestyle changes.

WHAT DO THE NUMBERS MEAN?

The results of your cholesterol test will come to your doctor in a series of numbers. Ask your doctor to obtain a copy for you as well; you won't see your report unless you specifically ask the doctor for a copy.

Applying those numbers to your own health situation, and using them to guide your lifestyle choices, can be confusing at first. We'll keep the information here as basic as possible to keep the confusion down—but it's important to understand what your test results mean so that you and your doctor *can* make the best choices for your healthier future.

Also, you will often see cholesterol measures shown as milligrams per deciliter of blood (mg/dL). To keep things simple, we will just use the numbers themselves in this book. In other words, when you read "120," it's the same as "120 mg/dL." We're just not using the scientific label.

In 2004, the NCEP determined the following guidelines for healthy LDL cholesterol, HDL cholesterol, triglycerides and total cholesterol levels:

LDL (Lousy) Cholesterol

LDL cholesterol is the one that clings to the insides of your arteries, eventually becoming atherosclerosis and forming plaque. Therefore, you want to aim for low numbers in this category. The size and type of LDL particles matter as well. We will discuss that in Chapter 3; for now we'll just focus on your test numbers and what they mean.

- 99 or lower is optimal; some doctors work with patients to get their LDL levels down to 70.

- 100–129 is considered "slightly higher than optimal." If your LDL level is in this range, there is no cause for alarm, but you should assess your risk factors and try to reach a lower level.

- 130–159 is rather high. If your LDL is in this range, you are at risk for heart disease and need to seriously consider lifestyle changes, at least, to lower your LDL level.

- 160–189 is in the high range. You are at risk for heart disease and should alert your doctor, if he isn't already aware, of your high reading. He will want to work with you to lower your LDL level as quickly as possible.

- Over 190 is a very high LDL measure. You are at high risk for heart disease. Chances are, your doctor will want to prescribe cholesterol-lowering medication (statins) to get your LDL lowered quickly.

HDL (Happy) Cholesterol

Picture a cat picking up her baby kitten between her teeth, carrying it across the yard and placing it where it belongs. That's what HDL cholesterol does for us—it snatches up the excess LDL cholesterol in our blood and takes it to our livers, where it will be disposed of. HDL helps us maintain low levels of LDL, so we want *high* numbers of HDL.

(If it's difficult to remember which is the "bad" cholesterol and which is "good," or which we want more of, just think of HDL = happy = high numbers, and LDL = lousy = low numbers.)

- Sixty and above signifies optimal HDL. The NCEP guidelines use 60 as the optimal measure for both men and women.

- The American Heart Association differentiates between the sexes, defining HDL of less than 50 as a risk factor for men, and HDL of less than 40 a risk factor for women. Talk with your doctor as to whether he or she agrees with the NCEP or the AHA.

Triglycerides

Triglycerides, a type of fat in your blood, are independent from cholesterol, but they work hand-in-hand with cholesterol and, if your levels are elevated, help to build a higher risk of heart disease. In women, very high triglyceride levels (above 500) signal another threat: inflammation of the pancreas, which can be life-threatening.

Excess triglycerides are created by excess body fat, too little exercise, diabetes, alcohol and some drugs, including estrogen, steroids and beta-blockers. They are most responsive to lifestyle changes, however, and show great improvement with moderate weight loss, exercise, and the kinds of healthy dietary changes you will read about in Chapters 4 and 5.

Triglyceride measures are the same for both men and women.

- 149 or less is considered normal.

- 150–199 is borderline, or slightly, high. If your triglycerides fall in this range, look at your lifestyle factors that might influence them—exercise, alcohol, body weight, body fat—and decide if you should alter them somewhat.

- 200–499 is high and puts you at risk for heart disease. Talk with your doctor about treatments or changes you should make.

- 500 and over is considered a very high triglyceride level. You and your doctor should devise a plan immediately for reducing the triglycerides in your blood.

Total Cholesterol

- 200 or less is considered low risk for heart disease.

- 200–239 is considered borderline or slightly high, and a score in this range puts you at slight risk for developing heart disease.

- Any total cholesterol score above 240 is considered high—but don't consider this figure alone in calculating your risk for heart disease. HDL, LDL and triglyceride levels all should be regarded separately.

If your total cholesterol level is above 240, you are hardly alone: About 17 percent of American adults, or almost one in five of us, have total cholesterol levels of 240 or more. The average is about 203, or slightly above the low-risk mark, though some ethnic groups, including African Americans, average at somewhat higher levels.

LEARN THE SYMPTOMS OF A HEART ATTACK!

You've heard these familiar heart attack symptoms:

• Chest pain (angina) that might come in waves, often feeling like something heavy is sitting on your chest or squeezing it.
• Pain in the stomach, back or arm.
• Getting tired very quickly during physical activity or exercise.
• Difficulty breathing.

Women, however, need to watch for a different set of symptoms, says a recent study by the National Institutes of Health. In fact, fewer than 30 percent of the women in their research reported feeling chest pain before their heart attacks; most of their symptoms were ordinary feelings that most women experience at times:

• Unusual fatigue.
• Sleep disturbance.
• Shortness of breath.
• Indigestion.
• Anxiety.

Extreme fatigue and sleep disturbance were the most widely reported symptoms. During their actual heart attacks, women also reported experiencing a cold sweat, weakness and dizziness.

The message: Pay attention to your body and its strong signals. Even if a symptom is an "ordinary" feeling, if it seems out of place or you can't think of a reason why you would be feeling that way, get help quickly.

YOU CAN'T CONTROL ALL OF YOUR RISK FACTORS

Your lipid profile is only one piece of the picture. A collection of factors work together to raise your cholesterol levels, including a few you can't control—your age, your gender and your heredity.

Like a lot of ailments and physical conditions, high cholesterol levels can be genetic—sometimes caused by a disorder we discussed briefly in Chapter 1, called familial hypercholesterolemia (FH). When FH strikes, LDL levels are elevated, occasionally even at birth, and can bring on an early heart attack.

Aside from such specific conditions, having males in the family who experienced heart disease when they were younger than fifty-five, or women with heart disease younger than sixty-five, is a strong enough history of coronary artery disease to say there is a genetic link. If you have such a family history of heart disease, be sure to check your cholesterol levels regularly.

Another risk that's out of your hands is your age. Not every mature person is at risk for having a heart attack, by any means—but if you are a man older than forty-five, or a woman over fifty-five, your risk of elevated cholesterol levels has increased since you were younger.

As for your sex, men generally have lower HDL cholesterol levels in their younger years than women, while women usually have lower LDL. But women lose their advantage once they reach fifty-five. Younger women in their childbearing years are "protected" somewhat by their high estrogen production, because estrogen raises HDL cholesterol levels. Once they reach menopause, however, women lose that protection and share the same age-related risk as men.

RISK FACTORS YOU *CAN* CONTROL

When you picked up this book to read, it was because you wanted to learn how to lower and regulate your cholesterol levels, or the levels of someone you care about. Many people find it possible to control their cholesterol naturally, without the help of medications, and they do it by managing these factors, all of which contribute to high cholesterol.

- *Your diet.* Doctors still are not certain just how eating large amounts of saturated fat produces excess cholesterol in your blood, but the two are strongly linked—and they are absolutely certain that high blood cholesterol causes atherosclerosis, or hardening or narrowing of the arteries, which leads to heart disease and heart attacks. Saturated fats, trans-fatty acids, and cholesterol from meat and cheese all contribute to high cholesterol.

- *Excess weight.* There is no debate: Obesity can reduce HDL cholesterol and increase LDL cholesterol, as well as increase the total cholesterol score.

- *Not enough exercise.* If you don't exercise regularly, and spend much of your day sitting, you are contributing to another risk factor for high cholesterol. If you begin a routine of deliberate, regular exercise, your LDL level will decrease and your HDL will rise.

- *Diabetes.* Diabetes in itself is a risk factor for heart disease, and it may contribute to unhealthy cholesterol levels. High LDL levels coupled with diabetes are a dangerous combination, putting you at high risk for coronary heart disease.

- *High blood pressure.* High cholesterol and high blood pressure are a highly unhealthy combination, dramatically increasing your risk of heart attack and heart disease. You cannot be heart-healthy with high blood pressure.

- *Smoking.* On its own, cigarette smoking is a risk factor for atherosclerosis and heart disease. It also may decrease HDL cholesterol.

The NCEP recommends that everyone get their cholesterol levels tested at least once every five years, even if they are not at risk for heart disease. If any of the above risk factors sounds familiar, your doctor may want you to be tested more often.

LOCATION, LOCATION, LOCATION

Apparently, where you live can affect your heart health, says a group of researchers for Kaiser Permanente in Oakland, California. They studied more than 46,000 people in northern California who had suffered heart attacks in the past decade and found that their rate of having a second heart attack had dropped by 24 percent in the past ten years. Moreover, the most severe types of heart attacks among that group dropped by 62 percent.

Scientists attributed the patients' improved rates to their targeting risk factors, including healthier blood pressure and cholesterol levels. Over the course of the study, those with healthy LDL cholesterol levels increased from 67 to 73 percent.

The findings don't reflect heart attack statistics in other regions of the country, but they do highlight the positive outcomes that are possible when we pay attention to risk factors. One vital note: All participants were fully insured by Kaiser Permanente, so they had access not only to treatment in the event of an emergency, but they also had received quality preventive care.

OKAY, MY RISK IS HIGH—NOW WHAT?

You've recognized the risk factors in yourself, or perhaps you've already been tested and discovered you have high cholesterol levels in your blood—an LDL score between 160 and 189—or even what's considered "moderately high," between 130 and 159. What's the next step?

You have many options. If your cholesterol levels are only moderately high, then you may be able to lower your LDL and triglycerides, and boost your HDL levels, with lifestyle changes. We will learn in later chapters how to develop heart-healthy cholesterol levels by implementing changes in your food, exercise, stress reduction, and dietary supplement routines.

The mission of this book is to help you manage your cholesterol naturally, if at all possible. For many Americans with high cholesterol, however, that may not be a realistic goal. Their physicians may want to prescribe statin medications for them.

If, on the other hand, your LDL and triglyceride levels are only slightly or moderately elevated, then you may be able to get them to a healthy level with diet and lifestyle changes. For some people, one facet of a healthy lifestyle is supplementation; a number of natural supplements have been proven to lower cholesterol levels for some people, and we've provided detailed information on many of them in Chapter 7, "Supplementing Your Wellness Plan."

WHAT'S YOUR HEART ATTACK RISK?

Would you like to know your chances of suffering a heart attack in the next ten years? Go to the National Cholesterol Education Program's website and use that agency's interactive "heart attack calculator" to find out: hp2010.nhlbihin.net/atpiii/calculator.asp?

usertype = pub. You will need to know your total cholesterol levels and your HDL cholesterol and systolic blood pressure numbers. Enter those, plus your age, gender, whether you are a smoker and whether you are on medication for high blood pressure, and click on the button that says, "Calculate Your 10-Year Risk." You will know immediately whether, statistically speaking, you are in a high-risk category for heart disease.

STATINS: WHEN LIFESTYLE CHANGE ISN'T ENOUGH

Statins, or HMG-CoA reductase inhibitors, are prescription drugs that treat high cholesterol; they work by slowing cholesterol production in the liver, and by helping to lure the LDL cholesterol to the liver to be excreted. Since an unhealthy diet and lack of exercise contribute to most cases of high cholesterol, many doctors prescribe statins along with a menu of lifestyle changes. Some patients will take the statins only for the short term, while many will continue taking the medications for life. Every case is different.

Examples of statins are:

- Atorvastatin (Lipitor®)
- Fluvastatin (Lescol®)
- Lovastatin (Mevacor®)
- Pravastatin (Pravachol®)
- Rosuvastatin (Crestor®)
- Simvastatin (Zocor®)

Statins are not without side effects, though most are minor: headache, dizziness, stomach upset and, according to new research reported in *Canadian Medical Association Journal,* myopathy (a disease involving damaged muscle fibers), myalgia (muscle aches) and possible muscle damage.

To avoid the more serious side effects, some holistic physicians recommend that patients taking statin medications also take Coenzyme Q_{10}, which can reduce muscle myopathy and other statin side effects. They also recommend supplementing with vitamin D, which helps build muscle tissue.

If your cholesterol levels are not in the "high" or "very high" range, you might want to try the more natural, drug-free approach—but if your doctor has prescribed a cholesterol-lowering drug, don't reject it without talking to him first. And if you do decide to try a more heart-healthy lifestyle instead of prescription meds, try the plan for three months, then ask your doctor to give you a new lipid panel test. If your cholesterol levels have not reduced at the end of your three-month trial period, take the statins.

And, it's important to note, *never* stop taking a drug too soon. If you take statin medications for a time and decide to try lowering your cholesterol levels with lifestyle changes alone, talk to your doctor about weaning you off the prescription drug in a healthy way. Many people who stop taking statins find that their cholesterol levels climb back up again over time and their risk of developing heart disease returns. For some, statins are a lifetime commitment, while others who have eliminated some of their serious heart disease risks, such as smoking and obesity, are able to *gradually* stop taking the medications. This is a decision you and your doctor should make together.

IS ASPIRIN THERAPY FOR YOU?

If your risk of heart disease is in the "high" range, with an LDL score higher than 160, some experts suggest that taking a "baby" or low-dose aspirin once a day can be an effective preventative because aspirin helps prevent clots from forming. It also fights inflammation, another factor in heart attacks. Aspirin, in fact, can help lower your heart attack risk by as much as 44 percent. It's also thought to lower your risk of colon, breast and prostate cancer by as much as 40 percent.

When doctors recommend taking aspirin for heart health, the usual regimen is two low-dose aspirin (or 165 mg total) per day with a full glass of warm water. The water is important, because 70 percent of aspirin-related side effects are caused by the aspirin's sticking to the stomach and intestinal lining and eroding it. All pills, in fact, should be downed with a full glass of water to prevent similar problems.

The effectiveness of an aspirin regimen, however, varies between men and women, and between age groups. Check with your doctor before you start, and be sure to check the dosage on the packaging before you take the aspirin for heart health. Some of the "quick-dissolve" are reported to contain several times the aspirin dosage recommended for heart health, and they may also contain caffeine. Again, discuss aspirin in general, and the brand and dosage you're planning to take, with your doctor.

TREAT YOUR HEART WITH TLC

Whether you decide on the natural approach to managing your cholesterol—with heart-healthy lifestyle changes—or take prescription medications, your doctor probably will recommend you look at your heart with TLC—not only Tender Loving Care (always a good idea), but with Therapeutic Lifestyle Changes.

TLC is the brainchild of the National Cholesterol Education Program (NCEP) of the National Heart, Lung, and Blood Institute (NHLBI) of the National Institutes of Health (NIH). It's a step-by-step plan to lowering cholesterol with reasonable physical activity, a heart-healthy diet, and managing other risk factors such as smoking and high blood pressure.

We will learn more about designing your own TLC program in Chapters 5, 6, and 7, where we discuss eating plans and exercise. First, in Chapter 3, you will want to know about other conditions affected by cholesterol; heart disease isn't the only consequence of having high cholesterol levels, by far.

Why else should you care about cholesterol, besides heart disease? We'll give you plenty of reasons.

CHAPTER THREE

It's Not All About Cholesterol

Cholesterol doesn't act alone in contributing to heart disease—in fact, half of all heart attacks happen in people with healthy cholesterol levels! Even if you've been vigilant about your heart health, had your cholesterol tested and found that your levels are all in the healthy range, you could have another condition, a severe risk factor, that influences how cholesterol behaves in your body and can increase your heart attack risk.

The most serious of these possibilities is systemic inflammation. It's important to understand inflammation, and in this chapter we will explain why, and describe the tests that can measure it. We're also going to describe additional tests that doctors can give beyond the standard lipid profile, and why they can be vital in revealing a fuller, more accurate picture of your true heart attack risk. (Not all doctors give these additional tests as a matter of routine, so you may need to ask for them.)

Lastly, we will look at links between heart disease and other conditions, primarily diabetes and osteoporosis.

INFLAMMATION—LIKE KINDLING FOR THE HEART

You know inflammation when you see it: after an injury, even one as minor as a bee sting, the injured spot becomes red, it often swells and feels warm to the touch, and it can hurt. What you're actually seeing is the effect of millions of white blood cells, coming to protect the injury and fight off infections—your immune system doing its job.

In that same way that the bee sting gets inflamed, inflammation plays a major role in the process when an artery is injured and clogged, leading to heart disease and heart attacks. Your body responds in the same way—but in this case, the "injury" is caused by oxidized LDL cholesterol, agitating and wearing a hole into the artery wall. The damage is aggravated if you smoke cigarettes, have high blood sugar or diabetes, or have high blood pressure. Your immune system sends white blood cells, called *monocytes*, to try and repair the damage: inflammation at work.

The monocytes cluster in the artery wall, where they transform into *macrophages*, or a slightly different type of white blood cell whose mission is to destroy unwelcome visitors such as bacteria, viruses or LDL cholesterol by eating them. They literally stuff themselves with the unwanted substance, then—just as many of us do after stuffing ourselves with a heavy Thanksgiving dinner—they line up along the artery wall and relax there.

The problem is, they hang out in our arteries indefinitely, forming a fatty streak along the wall. More LDL cholesterol comes along over the years, and the long corridor of fatstuffed macrophages hardens and turns into plaque.

We've talked about plaque forming in Chapter 1. Our arteries try to heal that, too, by covering the plaque with smooth muscle cells, forming a fibrous "cap"—but macrophages kill those newer cells, too, and the cap can rupture. A blood clot may then form around the rupture, plugging up the artery the rest of the way, and blood can no longer travel through the artery at all. When this happens, the outcome, after all of these attempts at healing, is a heart attack. And it all started with LDL cholesterol burrowing into the artery wall, and our immune system's inflammatory attempt at healing the wound. The more inflammation occurring in and around the plaque in our arteries, scientists believe, the greater our chances of having a heart attack.

INFLAMMATION MATTERS

Inflammation is considered by many scientists to be an important contributing cause of cancer, osteoarthritis and Alzheimer's disease, as well as heart disease. So, there's all the more reason to follow the advice later in this chapter on reducing inflammation in your body.

The fact is, if it continues for too long and we don't control it, inflammation can drive disease. A long-running infection from some condition totally apart from your coronary arteries—say, gum disease—can keep your immune system working hard for a long time, trying to fight that infection. That can't go on forever, and at some point your immune cells will lash out and attack the wrong cells, or the wrong part of the body.

When your body's efforts to fight infection go haywire in that way, what started as a healthy immune response becomes disease. Seemingly unrelated conditions, including multiple sclerosis, arthritis and even some cancers, as well as heart disease, have sometimes been attributed to an infection.

DENTAL INFLAMMATION AND YOUR HEART: THE CONNECTION IS REAL

You know that plaque buildup on your teeth isn't healthy, but you may not know the specific reasons why.

Dental plaque is sometimes referred to as a "biofilm"—a thin, sticky film composed of living bacteria that lives in your mouth. It forms constantly, all day long, covering your gum tissue, teeth, and dentures or crowns. It resists sugars and starches, so when you eat or drink something sweet or starchy, your plaque-bacteria sends out acids to attack the sugar and starch. Unfortunately, the acids also attack the enamel on your teeth.

And this plaque isn't just messy to the touch; it is so "sticky" that it holds onto those acids so they are adhering to your teeth and gums as long as the plaque is there. Eventually, the acids break down the enamel on your teeth, resulting in tooth decay.

When plaque builds up, it also can lead to several progressive gum diseases. The first would be gingivitis, which brings tender, swollen gums that often bleed when you brush your teeth. As it worsens, severe periodontal (gum) disease develops, in which your gum tissue can pull away from your teeth, enabling the bacteria to destroy the bone that supports your teeth.

But dental plaque is connected to health problems that appear beyond your mouth. Research has found strong links between gum diseases and diabetes, dementia, rheumatoid arthritis, premature birth and—importantly—heart disease. The one characteristic that all of these conditions share with periodontal disease is inflammation; the most prevalent theory is that bacteria from the mouth and gums can enter the bloodstream and infect other body organs and systems. And, scientists have found, heart disease and heart attacks are found more often in people with periodontal disease.

HOW DO YOU KNOW IF YOU HAVE HEART-RELATED INFLAMMATION?

Inflammation, you've read, can be a good thing. It is one of our body's clearest signals that we have an infection, an injury, or other condition that needs to be treated, such as arthritis or even cancer. How can we tell if some part of our body is experiencing inflammation? There is a simple test for it, measuring the amount of C-reactive protein, or CRP, in our blood.

CRP is produced by the liver and, in medical terms, is an "acute phase reactant." Simply put, that means we produce more of it as a response to inflammation, so that when inflammation is present, our CRP levels are higher.

CRP is not a risk factor for heart disease; rather, it *indicates* the possible presence of a risk factor. The distinction is important—as is the word "possible," as high levels of CRP in the blood also can indicate inflammation in other body systems besides cardiovascular. For that reason, a more refined measurement is used when your physician is specifically looking for arterial inflammation; that measure is referred to as hsCRP. Still, any inflammation in your body, even if it's unrelated to CRP—such as an arthritis flare-up—might show up as a higher-than-usual CRP level, so the Centers for Disease Control (CDC) advises taking two CRP tests, about two weeks apart.

CRP test results, according to the American Heart Association (AHA) and the CDC, are as follows:

- 1 milligram (mg) per liter or less indicates low risk for cardiovascular disease.

- 1 to 3 mg per liter indicates a moderate risk for heart disease.

- More than 3 mg per liter indicates a high risk for heart disease.

- Very high CRP levels (10 mg or higher) sometimes are present right after an acute plaque rupture in the artery, such as a heart attack or stroke.

Unlike cholesterol testing, which is recommended for all adults, the CDC doesn't advise CRP testing for everyone. Usually, CRP levels are viewed as supplemental information in testing whether a person is at cardiac risk, taken into account along with other factors such as smoking, high blood pressure, age, obesity and high cholesterol levels. If none of those risk factors are present, then most doctors will not test for CRP. Taken alone, it's not a reliable predictor of heart attacks or heart disease.

SHOULD EVERYONE TRY TO LOWER THEIR CRP?

Health authorities stop short of saying that everyone should work on lowering their CRP levels, especially since they may or may not indicate heart risk. *CRP is a better predictor of heart disease risk for women than for men.* A study performed by Brigham and Women's Hospital in Boston followed almost 28,000 healthy women for eight years. Researchers found a direct correlation between the women's CRP levels and their risk of heart attacks, strokes and other heart problems—more so, in fact, than measuring the women's LDL levels. Women with high CRP experienced twice as many episodes of heart disease as women with high LDL. Even more alarming: Women with a high CRP measurement and low LDL suffered more heart attacks than women with low CRP and high LDL. The bottom line is that women need to be aware of their CRP levels and, if they are high, adjust their lifestyles accordingly—even if their LDL levels are normal.

Whether you are a man or a woman, the experts do recommend adopting healthy practices that will make you healthier overall *and* have the incidental effect of lowering your CRP. These are straightforward changes that would benefit anyone, regardless of their CRP levels—and they are habits that you will read repeatedly in this book (but they bear repeating!):

- *If you smoke, stop smoking.* Smoking cigarettes elevates CRP levels, and quitting lowers them. It also cuts your risk of COPD, bronchitis, heart disease, stroke, and many cancers, including those of the lung, bladder, esophagus and mouth.

- *If you are overweight, bring your weight down to a healthy level.* People who carry excess pounds have higher CRP levels; losing as few as fifteen pounds also can lower LDL cholesterol (which we will talk about in later chapters about food and lifestyle changes), blood pressure and your risk of developing certain other conditions, such as diabetes.

- *If you don't exercise, begin now.* People who are physically fit generally have lower CRP levels, as well as lower risk of developing a multitude of other conditions, including depression.

ARE STATINS AN ANSWER?

What about statins for preventing heart disease, if your cholesterol is normal but your CRP is high? No discussion of CRP is complete without mentioning the famous JUPITER study, released in 2008, and the FDA's approval in February 2010 of Crestor, a popular statin drug, for preventing heart disease in some people (men over fifty years old and women older than sixty) who have high CRP levels and at least one other risk factor for heart disease, such as low HDL cholesterol, high blood pressure, a family history of premature heart disease, or smoking.

As you might imagine, the study results and subsequent FDA approval are controversial in the medical community.

The study was based on more than 18,000 individuals and funded by Crestor's manufacturer, AstraZeneca Plc. As *The New England Journal of Medicine* reported, the study subjects' risk of heart disease was 44 percent lower after using Crestor for less than two years. Some noted cardiologists object to giving a statin drug to patients as a "quick fix" for their heart disease risk factors, without the patients' first changing the lifestyles that put them at risk in the first place. Others point to possible side effects of statins, such as myalgia (severe muscle pain) and an increased risk of developing diabetes, as reasons not to prescribe statins unless they are necessary.

For now, statins remain an option for some patients with elevated CRP levels.

BEYOND THE LIPID PANEL

These are other tests you may want your doctor to give you.

LDL Particle Size

You have two varieties of LDL in your system: the small, dense particles and larger, fluffy particles. Whichever size dominates is determined by your genes—and, if you ever have a heart attack, it is the size of your LDL cholesterol that can tip the balance in terms of the damage done to your arteries. LDL particle size isn't always assessed when doctors measure cholesterol levels, but it's a good idea to ask your doctor if he or she would include a particle size test when your cholesterol is tested. About half of all men with coronary artery disease (CAD), and a third of premenopausal women with CAD will find high measures of small, dense LDL, according to the Centers for Disease Control. And, because all things work together in our bodies, it may not surprise you to learn that small, dense LDL is more common in people who carry excess weight, eat a high-carbohydrate diet and get little exercise.

Here's why LDL particle size matters. Imagine that you have two cups on the desk in front of you. One cup contains frozen peas, and the other contains frozen strawberries. Both cups weigh the same—yet, if you tip them onto their sides, the frozen strawberries will roll easily across the desk, while some of the peas will get stuck in the cracks of the desktop.

That's a simplistic view of the way small, dense LDL

particles—the peas—behave alongside the larger, puffier strawberry-LDL particles. Your LDL cholesterol levels might appear to be normal. But if your LDL is predominantly the smaller, denser type, then more of those particles will adhere to the walls of your arteries than if your LDL was mostly the larger, fluffy version. What's worse, small LDL particles tend to adhere to sugars, and people with small, dense LDL are at greater risk of developing diabetes sometime in their lives.

The good news: You *can* conquer your genes and transform small, dense LDL into the larger, fluffy, less harmful type. That all-important transformation happens when you make the lifestyle changes you will read about in the chapters to come—eating a heart-healthy diet, exercising regularly, and, if you choose, adding nutritional supplements to your daily routine.

LP(a), Little Troublemaker

Lipoprotein (a), called "lipoprotein little-a," is a particle that partners LDL fat with a chemical that interferes with our blood's clotting abilities. It's estimated that up to 30 percent of heart disease patients have Lp(a), and is especially prevalent in families with a history of early heart disease. Most often, Lp(a) is found in the plaque of patients with unstable heart disease.

Because Lp(a) has been found in such a large portion of people with heart disease—in some instances tripling their risk of CAD—and is often found in people with healthy LDL and HDL levels, some experts recommend that everyone be tested for Lp(a) when they have their initial cholesterol tests. With Lp(a), the number to watch for is 30: a test result showing less than 30 mg/dL of Lp(a) is considered healthy, while levels higher than 30 mg/dL indicated a risk of heart disease.

Unlike small-particle LDL and other heart risk factors, however, Lp(a) is stubborn—it does *not* respond to healthy lifestyle changes such as exercise and diet. But you can take these steps to bring your Lp(a) levels more in line.

- Consider taking niacin, one of the most popular dietary supplements for addressing high cholesterol levels. A daily dose of 500 to 2,000 milligrams can cut Lp(a) by 30 percent.

- L-carnitine, another nutritional supplement, can help lower Lp(a) levels by about 8 percent. You can read more about niacin and L-carnitine in Chapter 7, "Supplementing Your Wellness Plan."

- Walnuts, too, can bring down your Lp(a) levels by up to 6 percent. Eat about ten nuts each day, or a small handful—and watch the quantity. Nuts are packed with nutrients, but they also are high-calorie—and addicting!

HOMOCYSTEINE, THE PROTEIN-BUSTER

One more factor that can boost heart attack risk is homocysteine, an amino acid that forms as a by-product when we break down proteins from food—especially animal protein. When we have enough B vitamins in our system, we metabolize protein beautifully. Folic acid and vitamins B_6 and B_{12} are especially important to the process.

But when we don't get enough B vitamins, homocysteine levels become elevated—a situation strongly associated with heart disease and stroke risk.

Scientists are not sure whether homocysteine itself is the culprit or, like CRP, it's merely the indicator of other dangers. Some researchers speculate that it helps blood clots to form, harms arterial linings or even produces cancer-causing free radicals. Higher levels of homocysteine also have been connected to Alzheimer's disease and Parkinson's disease.

One thing is clear: High levels of homocysteine mean a

higher risk of heart disease. The number to aim for is 10 or lower micromoles per liter of blood—a healthy level. If your tests show 10 to 14 micromoles, your homocysteine is slightly elevated, and levels higher than 14 micromoles indicate a risk for heart disease and stroke.

In this instance, nutritional changes help immensely. The first step often suggested by health care professionals is a folic acid dietary supplement (the amount varies between specialists, but 400 mcg daily is recommended by many manufacturers). Among the foods known for their folic acid content are lettuce, asparagus, cabbage, oranges, strawberries, melons and whole grains.

Many doctors also recommend their patients cut back on their consumption of meat, dairy, caffeine and alcohol. And if the person is experiencing unusual stress, some exercise and stress-reducing techniques can help as well. (Read Chapter 8, "Lowering Cholesterol with Exercise," for a selection of exercises and relaxation techniques that can boost heart health.)

LOOK IN YOUR MEDICINE CABINET

Very few medications come with no side effects. Unfortunately, a medicine that's designed to resolve one problem sometimes contributes to another. For example, certain medications do elevate cholesterol and/or triglyceride levels as a side effect. Usually, the increase is small, but if you have other risk factors for heart disease, you may wish to discuss alternatives to the following medications with your doctor:

- *Steroids.* Allergies, asthma and several other conditions are sometimes treated with steroids, which are linked to slight increases in triglyceride and total cholesterol levels.

- *Progestin.* A component of birth control pills, progestin can raise LDL levels and lower HDL cholesterol.

In spite of that tendency, it has not been found to increase risk of heart disease.

• *Retinoids.* The problem with retinoids, used in treating acne and other skin problems, is that they contain
vitamin A, which can affect the liver—the producer
of cholesterol. Retinoids can raise cholesterol levels
slightly.

• *Beta blockers.* Rather than elevating cholesterol levels, beta blockers (used for treating high blood pressure) can boost triglycerides and the production of
other blood fats in a small percentage of people.

• *Diuretics.* No one knows why, but diuretics can cause
elevated triglyceride levels.

WHAT IS METABOLIC SYNDROME,
AND SHOULD I WORRY ABOUT IT?

Doctors often point to a phenomenon called "metabolic syndrome," sometimes called "insulin resistance." It's not a disease in itself; rather, it is a collection of risk factors which, if
they appear simultaneously in your system, work together to
greatly enhance your chances of developing heart disease
and type 2 diabetes—it can even double your risk!

When you have metabolic syndrome, it means that your
body no longer uses its insulin, which is produced by your
pancreas, efficiently. When insulin is used efficiently, it is the
agent that converts the glucose (sugar) in your blood into energy. But if insulin isn't used properly, it overloads your system and results in symptoms such as lethargy, weight gain,
and eventually type 2 diabetes and heart disease.

It's a bigger problem than researchers once realized: Today, because of the obesity epidemic in the U.S., it's estimated that about 25 percent of all American adults have
metabolic syndrome.

You have metabolic syndrome if you can claim at least three of these five risk factors:

1) *Belly fat.* Abdominal obesity is a much clearer indicator of heart disease than fat that you might carry in other parts of your body. Experts define it as a waist size of more than 40 inches for men and 35 inches for women.

2) *High blood sugar.* This is defined as higher than 100 to 125 milligrams per deciliter (mg/dL) when measured while fasting.

3) *High triglycerides.* For purposes of detecting metabolic syndrome, high triglycerides are defined as levels of 150 mg/dL or higher.

4) *Low HDL.* A lower "good" cholesterol level of 40 mg/dL for men, or 50 mg/dL for women, qualifies as a risk factor for metabolic syndrome.

5) *High blood pressure.* Blood pressure is measured in terms of systolic, referring to the contractions of the heart, over diastolic, referring to the rhythmic expansion of the heart's cavities as they fill with blood. The measurement is expressed as mm/Hg, or millimeters of mercury. If your measures are 130 systolic or higher, or 85 diastolic or higher, then your blood pressure is high enough to be a risk factor for metabolic syndrome.

The best remedy for metabolic syndrome, experts agree, is straightforward but not simple: Lose your excess weight. If you already have unhealthy cholesterol levels as part of your metabolic syndrome, they might require medication at first, to get them to a healthy level more quickly.

A change in diet and an exercise regimen will help to eliminate the belly fat, while at the same time lowering your

LDL and raising your HDL cholesterol, and reducing your CRP·(inflammation) scores. We'll look at programs and foods to help make that happen in Chapters 5 and 6, and learn about exercise and other healthy practices in Chapter 8.

And the news does get better. A study reported in the March, 2010 issue of *Circulation: Journal of the American Heart Association*, found that for obese people who lose weight, atherosclerosis can be reversible. The study was conducted in Israel, where doctors investigated whether overweight participants (mostly men) who followed three diets—the Mediterranean diet, a low-carbohydrate diet, and a low-fat diet—and added exercises to their routines could improve their cholesterol levels.

Participants following all three diets lost weight (an average of 11.7 pounds over two years), improved their HDL levels, lowered their blood pressure and decreased their average carotid vessel-wall volume and carotid artery thickness. Researchers concluded that the specific nutrients of the diets didn't influence the improvement in cholesterol levels, so much as the weight loss itself.

CHOLESTEROL AND "UNRELATED" CONDITIONS

Cholesterol is a fascinating reminder that every system in our bodies depends on every other system, and they all affect one another in real ways.

Some health conditions may appear to be isolated from cholesterol, but in reality they are influenced by your HDL, LDL and triglyceride levels. In some instances, high cholesterol levels even increase your risk of having these diseases, too. If you experience any of these, be sure to have your cholesterol levels checked.

- *Diabetes.* Glucose (sugar) clings to lipoproteins and the LDL is literally sugar-coated, enabling it to easily stick to artery walls and become plaque. People with diabetes often have high triglyceride and low

HDL levels, greatly increasing their risk of cardio-vascular disease.

• *High blood pressure.* When cholesterol hardens into plaque and narrows the arteries, the heart has to work much harder to pump blood through the smaller openings, causing blood pressure to rise.

• *Peripheral artery disease.* This condition refers to plaque-related narrowing in the arteries of the legs. The result is poor circulation, leg pain (especially when walking) and resistance to healing when there is a wound.

• *Cerebrovascular disease.* This phrase refers to both blockages in arteries of the brain, causing strokes.

• *Osteoporosis.* Researchers are still studying the relationship between osteoporosis and cholesterol, but a study of 2,500 postmenopausal women resulted in a quadrupled risk of heart attack among mature women with osteoporosis. Some experts believe the connection is related to a chronic vitamin D deficiency; some studies also have found greater levels of both coronary plaque and osteoporosis in people with low levels of vitamin D.

• *Alzheimer's disease.* In 2009, a thirty-year study concluded that high cholesterol and Alzheimer's are linked: Those middle-aged men and women with high total cholesterol levels (above 240 mg/dL) were 66 percent more likely to have Alzheimer's later in life than those with healthy (200 mg/dL or lower) levels. Those with borderline-high levels (200 to 239 mg/dL) showed a 52 percent higher risk. Higher cholesterol levels, researchers found, hinder the brain's ability to use glucose, which fuels the brain for normal functioning.

NOW, FOR YOUR HEALTHIER FUTURE

Understanding cholesterol and how it relates to heart disease, assessing your risk and being aware of how cholesterol affects other conditions build an essential foundation to creating a heart-healthy lifestyle.

Congratulations—you've completed that important phase! Now it's time to move on to the core of the book: actually creating your new, healthier life. We'll start with learning about food, what's healthy and what isn't, and then we'll take action: making the best food choices, strategizing about how to eat healthy in real-life situations like parties and dining out, and taking food supplements that can lower your cholesterol levels. Finally, we'll look at exercise and reducing stress, so that you can lose any excess weight and get even closer to your heart-healthy goals.

PART II

Creating a Healthier You

CHAPTER FOUR

You Are What You Eat

If this is the first book you've read about cholesterol, then the first section should have given you a fairly solid understanding of what it is, how it's measured and how it affects your health.

Now, you will start learning how to use that information to create a healthy lifestyle that will bring your own cholesterol levels in line. A number of lifestyle factors contribute to optimal cholesterol levels, and by far the most important of them is food—what you eat, how much you eat and your weight.

Food matters, and in this chapter you will learn why. More than half a century of research brings us evidence we can rely on, about fats (helpful and harmful), carbohydrates (refined vs. unrefined), and the impact of fiber, the glycemic index and sodium. This is the chapter that presents the science behind the latest nutritional advice from the experts.

Then, in Chapter 5, you will learn how to put those findings to good use, building an eating plan that will help you prevent cardiovascular disease (CVD)—particularly those cardio conditions involving high cholesterol. We'll take what we learn a step further in Chapter 6, applying that information to the real-life situations that can tempt us, confuse us and cause us to forget our wellness programs: shopping, entertaining and dining out. Chapter 7 provides mini-profiles of a long list of nutritional supplements, all of which can be helpful in reducing heart disease risk. Finally, Chapter 8 completes your heart-healthy lifestyle program with a host of exercise, relaxation, meditation and other lifestyle options that will help you to reach your goals.

EATING FOR HEART HEALTH

No doubt you've read plenty about the dangers of eating too much fat, sugar and sodium, especially in regard to heart health. What you don't read about so often is what you *should* eat to help you lower your cholesterol levels. But researchers at the Stanford Prevention Research Center, among others, have stated that eating well—not just avoiding certain foods—can be every bit as beneficial as focusing on the negative.

They proved their point by comparing two different low-fat diets. One of the diets kept the fat content to a minimum but didn't specify which types of foods participants should eat. They were permitted processed foods such as frozen waffles and turkey bologna sandwiches, along with low-fat prepared foods such as frozen lasagna and high-sugar (but low-fat) snacks.

The second group's low-fat diet was abundant in vegetables, fruits, whole grains and beans—all plant-based foods. The results were startling: Researchers had expected both groups to emerge with lowered cholesterol, which they did—but those who followed the plant-based diet enjoyed twice the decrease in LDL cholesterol (a 9.4 percent reduction, compared to a 4.6 percent reduction in the first group). No significant difference in HDL cholesterol or triglyceride levels was found.

The study makes a good case for the American Heart Association (AHA) guidelines, which recommend at least five daily servings of vegetables and fruit and at least six servings of grains—whole grains if possible. What's more, a person need not be a vegetarian to incorporate these amounts of plant-based foods into their lives. A "serving" of vegetables, for instance, is generally half a cup—and try using just half a cup of spinach or mixed greens in a salad! You will read more in Chapter 5 about easy ways to make health foods the foundation of your eating plan; for now you can just look at the evidence and, hopefully, begin to realize that the lifestyle changes required for heart health really aren't so difficult to make.

FATS AND OTHER NUTRIENTS THAT AFFECT YOUR HEART HEALTH

It almost seems as if we can't live with 'em and can't live without 'em—fats, that is. But you do need some fats in your system. For one thing, healthy fats (and you will read, later in this section, which fats are "healthy") give you energy. You also need fats because some nutrients—particularly vitamins A, D, E and K—are fat-soluble and can only be absorbed through fats.

Cholesterol, soluble fiber, stanols, sterols—these are all terms you hear bandied about when nutritionists promote healthy eating, but they don't always explain what these nutrients mean, especially in terms of how they affect cholesterol levels and heart health. Here, then, are the essentials.

Monounsaturated fats. These are the "healthy fats" that help to lower your blood cholesterol levels. Sometimes called alpha-linolenic acids or MUFAs (monounsaturated fatty acids), they're found in flax seeds, canola oil, olive oil, grapeseed oil and soy.

- *Relation to heart health:* Foods containing MUFAs are proven to reduce LDL cholesterol and may raise HDL cholesterol.
- *Recommendation:* The AHA recommends that most of your dietary fats be monounsaturated.

Polyunsaturated fats. These fats typically are liquid at room temperature and when refrigerated; they're found in nuts, some vegetable oils (soybean, corn, safflower oils) and fatty fish such as salmon, herring and trout.

- *Relation to heart health:* These fats can be beneficial to heart health when consumed in moderation; they are definitely preferable to saturated fat or trans fats. The healthiest type of polyunsaturated fats are called omega-3 fats sometimes called, "omega-3 fatty acids," and they are discussed in their own section below.
- *Recommendation:* Don't be afraid to eat polyunsaturated fats in moderation.

Omega-3 fats. Omega-3s are a form of polyunsaturated fats that not only are essential, but they are just about the healthiest polyunsaturated fat. We can't produce them ourselves, so we have to get them from food, primarily fish.

- *Relation to heart health:* Omega-3 fats can help lower cholesterol and triglyceride levels. They also decrease risk of arrhythmias and lower blood pressure slightly.
- *Recommendation:* The AHA recommends at least two servings of fatty fish each week—salmon, sardines, albacore tuna, mackerel and lake trout. They add that while it's preferable to get your omega-3s from food, people with coronary artery disease and those with high triglyceride levels might consider taking fish oil supplements.

Saturated fats. Usually solid at room temperature and in the refrigerator, these fats are mostly from animals: poultry with skin, whole-milk dairy products (butter, whole-fat cream cheese) and fatty meats and lard. Palm and coconut oil, although vegetable in origin, also are high in saturated fat.

- *Relation to heart health:* Foods containing saturated fats raise your blood cholesterol levels and increase your risk of heart disease. Many contain dietary cholesterol, which makes them even more unhealthy.
- *Recommendation:* The AHA recommends that saturated fats account for no more than 7 percent of your daily intake. So, if you're on a 2,000-calorie-per-day diet, that's only about 140 calories, or the equivalent of one glass of whole milk or 1½ tablespoons of butter.

Trans fats. Also called trans fatty acids, trans fats are found in "hydrogenated" foods, or foods to which hydrogen was added, to keep them solid: margarine, cookies, donuts and foods fried in hydrogenated shortening are examples. We also find them in highly processed foods.

- *Relation to heart health:* Trans fats raise your bad (LDL) cholesterol and lowers your good (HDL) cholesterol. Eating trans fats boosts your risk of developing heart disease and type 2 diabetes.
- *Recommendation:* Of all the fats, *trans fats are the worst and should be avoided.* In the supermarket, look for "hydrogenated fats" or "partially hydrogenated fats" on nutrition labels; those are trans fats. The AHA recommends that trans fats amount to no more than 1 percent of your daily fat intake. You'll read more about trans fats in Chapter 6 where we discuss "healthy shopping."

Carbohydrates. We get the most of our energy from carbohydrates, and they should comprise about 60 percent of our daily intake. Most carbohydrates, or "carbs," come from plant sources; we know them mostly as sugars and starches. Carbohydrates are either simple or complex.

Simple carbs supply quick, short-term energy but few other nutrients, if any. The most common of these is glucose, found naturally in many fruits and vegetables, also produced in the body as we break down other foods. We also find simple carbs in white bread and foods made with enriched flour.

Complex carbs supply longer-lasting energy, plus nutrients and fiber. We find complex carbohydrates in whole grains; beans and peas; and tubers such as potatoes and yams.

- *Relation to heart health*: Foods made largely of simple carbs, such as white bread, pasta and sweets, are high on the glycemic index, which you will read about later in this chapter. They cause your blood sugar to spike; women who eat those foods regularly are more than twice as likely to develop heart disease as women who rarely eat them.
- *Recommendation:* Eat foods made of complex carbs as much as possible; choose them over simple carbs whenever you can.

Soluble and insoluble fiber. Fiber is a form of carbohydrate. Soluble fiber is found in oats, rice bran, barley, apples, citrus fruit and strawberries. Insoluble fiber appears in cabbage, carrots, beets, Brussels sprouts, cauliflower, wheat cereals and whole-wheat breads.

- *Relation to heart health:* Soluble fiber is proven to lower blood cholesterol levels. Though insoluble fiber does not lower blood cholesterol, it is important to healthy colon function.

- *Recommendation:* Choose whole-grain and fiber-rich foods whenever possible.

Sugars. Sugars are sweeteners. In our bodies, they appear most commonly as glucose, which, if not used for energy, is stored as fat.

- *Relation to heart health:* Added sugars are directly linked to obesity, hypertension (high blood pressure) and other risk factors for CVD and CAD, including cholesterol levels.
- *Recommendation:* The AHA recommends that women limit their sugar consumption to 100 calories per day, and men limit theirs to 150 calories.

Sodium. Sodium can be added or occur naturally; it's found in table salt, baking soda and some medicines, including many over-the-counter remedies such as antacids.

- *Relation to heart health:* A high-sodium diet contributes to elevated blood pressure, thereby increasing the risk for heart disease.
- *Recommendation:* Because of new findings, the AHA revised its guidelines regarding sodium in January 2010, and now recommends that Americans limit their sodium intake to 1,500 mg per day.

Carotenoids. This is the substance that gives yellow and orange plant foods their appealing colors. Some pink animal foods, such as salmon and shrimp, also contain carotenoids.

- *Relation to heart health:* The presence of carotenoids in food signals that the food helps to lower cholesterol levels, as well as preventing *ischemic* (resulting from a blood clot) stroke. There's even evidence that they help prevent some cancers.

- *Recommendation:* Experts advise getting at least one serving of carotenoids every day. They're found in carrots, pumpkins and other yellow and orange fruits and veggies, and the seafoods mentioned above. If you follow the National Cholesterol Education Program (NCEP) recommendation of two to four servings of fruits and three to five servings of vegetables every day, you're sure to get the carotenoids you need.

Alcohol. For our purposes, "alcohol" refers to alcoholic beverages—wine, beer and spirits.

- *Relation to heart health:* Some research suggests that antioxidants and other ingredients in red wine may contribute to higher levels of "good" cholesterol, HDL, in the blood.
- *Recommendation:* The AHA recommends that if you drink alcohol, do so in moderation: one glass of wine or beer per day for women, and two glasses for men. However, the NCEP advises that, if you don't drink now, it's wise not to start.

Now that you have the most updated recommendations for consuming these most common nutrients, what follows are several interesting examples of recent research into food and heart health.

BUSTING MYTHS ABOUT SATURATED FATS

A 2010 study by the Harvard School of Public Health has challenged the tried-and-true assumption about the evils of saturated fats.

Researchers found that risks of coronary heart disease

(CHD) and cardiovascular disease (CVD) were not elevated by the subjects' saturated fat intake per se, but that the converse was true: Replacing saturated fats with polyunsaturated or monounsaturated fats did lower both LDL and HDL cholesterol levels.

The study also found that replacing saturated fats with increased carbohydrates, especially dense or "simple" carbs, increased the risk factors for the metabolic syndrome that we're all trying to avoid—increased triglycerides, small LDL particles and reduced HDL cholesterol levels. The recommendation, for now, continues to be that we should eat animal fats in moderation and, at the same time, limit our simple carbohydrates.

NEW FINDINGS ON FIBER

A new, major study out of Harvard University, published in the journal *Circulation* in May 2010, underscores the importance of dietary fiber in fighting heart disease. After following almost 8,000 nurses over age thirty with type 2 diabetes for nearly three decades, researchers found that the women who ate the most bran-rich, high-fiber whole grains showed a 35 percent lower risk of death from heart disease and a 28 percent lower risk of death from all causes—an important finding because people with diabetes overall have two to three times the risk of dying early from heart disease.

HOW IMPORTANT IS TOTAL FAT INTAKE?

One extraordinarily large study, the Women's Health Initiative, brought together nearly 49,000 postmenopausal women to fine-tune what we know about fats: that the kind of fats we eat matters a great deal in regard to cardiovascular disease (CVD).

Study participants, all women aged fifty to seventy-nine years, enrolled in forty clinics across the U.S. and follow-up

lasted for just over eight years. One group received only educational materials regarding diet; the other were coached
in intensive behavioral changes to reduce their total fat intake to 20 percent of calories and increase their vegetable
and fruit intake (five servings per day) and daily grains (six
servings).

The result: Although the group who received the training
did cut their fat consumption by more than 8 percent, there
was no significant difference between the groups regarding
the percentages who contracted heart disease. However, those
who ate fewer saturated fats or trans fats, or who boosted
their intake of vegetables and fruits, did show a trend toward
more reductions in heart disease risk. So, lowering total fat
consumption may not reduce your risk of CHD, stroke or
CVD, even if you eat more vegetables, fruits and grains. But
focusing on eating fewer saturated and trans fats, while eating more fruits, vegetables and grains, could offer significant
protection against heart disease in older women. Research
into the relationship between heart disease and healthy eating is ongoing

MORE DATA ON HEALTHY FATS

The OmniHeart diet, whose clinical trial was published in
the *Journal of the American Medical Association* (JAMA)
in 2005, further explored the question of which fats were
healthiest. Participants in the OmniHeart study, all of whom
had been diagnosed with mild hypertension, followed three
different diets—one high in carbohydrates, one high in protein and the third high in unsaturated fat. All of the diets
provided an abundance of fruits, vegetables and whole grains,
nonfat or low-fat dairy, and only lean meat cuts and skinless
poultry.

The results were surprising. The high-protein and high-
unsaturated fat diets both resulted in healthier cholesterol
levels and blood pressure measures than the high-carb
DASH diet, another eating plan that was popular at the time.

The message: Again and again, we're seeing that unsaturated fats, whole grains and fiber are the building blocks of heart health.

YOUR GLYCEMIC LOAD, AND WHY YOU NEED TO CARE

You've read about the ways in which sugar, and a healthy blood sugar level, can affect your heart health—especially for those who are at risk of diabetes, because diabetes is a huge heart attack risk.

And you understand how carbohydrates are converted to glucose, or sugar, and either expended for energy, or stored as fat. The *glycemic index* is the measure that we use to determine how quickly a food becomes sugar. The idea is to look for low-glycemic foods, because they don't elevate your sugar levels. If a food has a high *glycemic load*, it quickly becomes sugar in the liver. The pancreas produces insulin to escort the sugar into the cells, where it might be used for energy. But with too many foods carrying a high glycemic load, those sugary calories get stored as fat—which, we already know, is a threat to heart health.

This is why people concerned with their cholesterol levels must be wary of a diet high in simple carbohydrates. If you consume too many simple carbs, loading up on white potatoes, breads and pasta, you could be contributing to abdominal fat and, eventually, higher cholesterol levels. Carbohydrates *should* be a major part of your diet—as long as they are complex carbs, like those you get from whole grains and vegetables.

MORE ON CARBOHYDRATES:
EMBRACE THEM—WITH CAUTION!

It's understandable that fats would take the front seat in any discussion of cholesterol. After all, it's the lipids that line your arteries and eventually harden into plaque, becoming atherosclerosis. Fats are the most obvious threat in the fight against heart disease, so we talk about them a lot.

But controlling carbohydrates is an important part of controlling your weight—and, hence, controlling your cholesterol levels—so you need to factor them into your new, healthy lifestyle.

You will find very few carbohydrates in animal products—that's one reason why being a vegetarian is no guarantee of being thin! The term "carbohydrates," as you read in the primer above, encompasses sugars and starches, which fuel us with energy, and fiber, which keeps us cleaned-out and regular. Just as there are different kinds of fats that behave differently in our bodies, however, likewise there are different kinds of carbohydrates—and their differences are just as important. This message was included briefly in the primer, but it's critical to a heart-healthy eating plan, so we are expanding it a bit here.

You already understand that your body will respond differently to 10 grams of trans fats—say, from eating French fries—than it would to 10 grams of unsaturated fats from a spoonful of olive oil. With carbohydrates, you need only concern yourself with two varieties—complex or slow-absorbing carbs, and simple or fast-absorbing carbs.

It's the simple, fast-absorbing carbs you want to keep to a minimum. They are the carbohydrates found in sugars and "dense," low-fiber breads and pastas. They will cause your blood glucose levels to spike, your insulin levels to go out of control, your belly to expand and, for some people, metabolic syndrome to develop.

At the end of Chapter 5, you will find a "nutrition counter" of nutrients found in foods commonly used in home cooking. (A similar counter of nutrients in popular restaurant meals follows Chapter 6.) In every category, you will see a wide disparity in the counts listed beside various food items. Chapter 5 is where we will start learning how to plan heart-healthy meals; for now, just remember that carbohydrates are important to weight control and should be in the front of your mind as you choose your foods and beverages.

Sugar and enriched white flour are the major carbohydrate culprits. A few examples of high-carb foods, dense with simple carbs or sugars, to eat in moderation:

- 1 cinnamon-raisin bagel = 31 carbohydrates
- White enriched-bread pita, 1 piece = 33 carbohydrates
- Cooked macaroni, enriched, 1 cup = 43 carbohydrates
- Cranberries, dried and sweetened, 1 cup = 102 carbohydrates
- Cola, 1 can, 16 fl. oz. = 51 carbohydrates

Complex carbohydrates, or the slow-absorbing kind, have a more complex cellular structure and include complex starches and fiber. A few examples:

- Oat bran, cooked, 1 cup = 25 carbohydrates
- Almonds, 1 cup = 20 carbohydrates
- Butternut squash, cooked, 1 cup = 22 carbohydrates
- Apple, raw w/skin, 3.25" diameter = 31 carbohydrates
- Chamomile tea, brewed, 1 cup = - carbohydrates

You'll notice that some of the complex carbohydrate foods, such as the apple, are relatively high in carbs. But when you view the entire nutrition profile of the foods, you will see that the apple contains only 23 grams of sugar, while the cup of dried cranberries carries a whopping 81 grams!

A CLOSER LOOK AT SUGAR

Do you crave dessert every night? Are you one of those people who thinks a deep-fried Mars bar would be a perfect ending to a meal?

If so, you've finally found something you can blame on your parents—at least a little bit.

Our genes were designed to help us survive in our environment, scientists say. We had to catch or grow our food, and it gave us fuel for the hard work we did every day. In these modern times, however, many of us don't work our bodies hard enough to burn the calories—the energy—that we feed ourselves. We don't need to climb hills, build shelters, plant crops and skin animals in order to survive.

Instead, in our "new" environment we drive to an air-conditioned supermarket and buy a pint of Ben & Jerry's to top off our meal of precooked, frozen, breaded veal cutlets and frozen broccoli in cream sauce—but we're still hard-wired to gorge and store all the calories we can. That's especially true of fats and sugars, which convert easily into fat for storage. So our sugar-filled, calorie-dense meals are stored, contributing to abdominal fat and inflammation associated with heart disease, diabetes, high blood pressure, strokes, joint problems, liver disease and even cancer.

Makes you want to stop what you're doing and go for a brisk walk, doesn't it?

In April 2010, JAMA published a study conducted by research at the Emory School of Medicine and Centers for Disease Control and Prevention in Atlanta, which looked at added sugars consumed and blood fat levels in 6,100 subjects. By "added sugars," we mean table sugar, honey and sugars in processed foods and drinks—candies, pastries, soft drinks, iced tea and canned fruits. Sugars that already existed in fruits and fruit juices didn't count.

Researchers found that added sugars accounted for more than 320 calories a day, on average, or 21.4 teaspoons! That's about 16 percent of the calories participants take in every day, compared to 11 percent in 1977. What's more, those who consumed the most sugar maintained the lowest HDL or "good" cholesterol levels, and the highest levels of triglycerides.

RESEARCHERS LOOK AT YOUR FAVORITE FOODS

In the last several years, as obesity (along with heart disease) has become epidemic in this country, researchers have stepped up their efforts to zero in on the causes and remedies for unhealthy cholesterol levels. They've uncovered some fascinating data regarding our most popular foods.

- It's been affirmed that eating nuts can help lower LDL cholesterol and triglyceride levels, but the most dramatic effects are seen in thin people, those who don't practice healthy eating habits, and those who began the study with high LDL and triglyceride levels. Conclusions from a pool of 25 studies in seven countries, released in May 2010 in *Archives of Internal Medicine*, showed that eating about 1½ ounces of nuts every day reduced LDL cholesterol levels, and elevated HDL levels, regardless of whether the subjects' LDL and HDL levels were healthy or unhealthy at the beginning of the studies. However, eating nuts only affected the triglyceride levels of people whose levels were unhealthy at the outset; the triglyceride levels of those who began the study with healthy triglycerides were not influenced by eating the nuts.

- In several different studies over the last decade, eating moderate amounts of walnuts, almonds, peanuts, hazelnuts, pecans, pistachios and some pine nuts also were found to help lower bad LDL cholesterol by as much as 10 percent, decrease triglycerides by more than 11 percent, and raise good HDL cholesterol by more than 5 percent, according to a study published in *The Journal of Nutrition*.

- However, not all nuts are created equal when it comes to improving cholesterol levels. Brazil nuts, macadamia nuts, cashew nuts and some types of pine nuts are not recommended by the FDA for improving cholesterol levels because of their high fat content. Still, they hastened to add, smaller amounts of these more fatty nuts can be beneficial to cholesterol levels, too.

- A recent study conducted at Harvard University found that coffee drinkers were less likely to die from heart-related diseases than nondrinkers. It protects against other diseases as well: a Norwegian study concluded that one serving of black coffee contains more anti-oxidants than a serving of raspberries, blueberries or pineapples. However, people concerned about their cholesterol levels should drink coffee brewed through a paper filter or instant coffee; unfiltered coffee—the type made in a French press—contains higher amounts of cafestol, a cholesterol-boosting substance.

- Cheese can be good for your cholesterol levels: A recent study at Wake Forest University School of Medicine in Winston-Salem, North Carolina, found that women who ate a serving of cheese every day (equal to the size of about four dice) had higher HDL and lower LDL levels than those who ate less cheese. Men who ate the same amount of cheese didn't fare as well, possibly because they chose cheeses containing more saturated fat and salt.

- Whole milk might be good for cholesterol levels, in spite of its high saturated fat and cholesterol content. Two studies published in the July 2010 issue of *The American Journal of Clinical Nutrition* (AJCN) found that women milk drinkers had a 26 percent lower risk of heart attacks. One theory, which researchers will continue to study, is that milk might lead to heart-healthier outcomes because it contains conjugated linoleic acid, or CLA.

- Dark chocolate can help keep your arteries wide open: researchers in Zurich, Switzerland tested heart transplant recipients two hours after they ate dark chocolate, and found their coronary artery diameters had increased significantly.

- Guacamole is a high-calorie treat, but it can help lower cholesterol levels. Eating avocados every day can reduce total cholesterol—but just a 2-tablespoon serving packs 5 grams of fat and 55 calories. Still, that's much healthier than the same amount of butter or mayonnaise, which contain 22 fat grams and 200 calories.

- Good news for wine drinkers—red wine directly affects blood fats in a healthy way! A study published in the July 2010 issue of *AJCN* found that resveratrol, a healthy ingredient in red wine, inhibits the growth of *preadipocytes*, or immature fat cells, into fully developed *adipocytes*, or fat cells. Furthermore, it suppressed the formation of inflammatory compounds. The research continues; scientists want to know whether this influence by resveratrol on fat cells might affect the risk of obesity and, consequently, heart disease risk.

- Even beer has some health benefits! It may be the last "food item" you would expect to see on a heart-healthy diet, but beer actually can contribute to heart health. We already knew beer was fat-free and cholesterol-free. Now, researchers at the University of Texas Southwestern Medical Center found in March 2010 that drinking one to two 12-ounce glasses of beer per day can reduce your risk of developing heart disease by up to 40 percent, even compared to people who never drink alcohol at all! They also found it can cut your risk of a stroke by 20 percent. One reason, they surmise, might be that beer contains vitamin B_6, which helps prevent homocysteine—an amino acid linked to heart disease—from accumulating. The scientists caution you to drink in moderation, especially because other studies show that drinking two or more glasses of alcohol per day, in any form, can increase a woman's chances of

developing breast cancer. *(Note: We are NOT recom-
mending that anyone drink two glasses of beer a
day, especially if you want to lose weight. You might
consider adding a small amount to your diet if you
want to gain weight; if not, a B-vitamin complex supplement is an alternative that might provide the same
heart-health benefits.)* And, of course, never drink
and drive.

NOW, WHAT TO DO ABOUT YOUR CHOLESTEROL?

This is the science—the up-to-date information that research
has given us about cholesterol. So how do we apply all of
this to our lives?

We begin with a healthy food plan. The NCEP has de-
vised an easy-to-follow, heart-healthy program, aptly called
TLC—Therapeutic Lifestyle Changes. TLC encompasses
healthy eating, exercise and stress reduction. We'll look at
the TLC approach to food in the next chapter, as well as
other heart-healthy diet plans.

The first four chapters gave you all the background you
need to understand why it's vital to lower your unhealthy cholesterol levels. Now, get set to begin your new heart-healthy
future!

CHAPTER FIVE

Your TLC Eating Plan

This is the point at which many people, as they read about eating for better health, fear that they'll have to start preparing all of their meals with a salad spinner.

Not so! You will see, as you read through this chapter, that healthy eating can be tastier and more satisfying than stuffing yourself with greasy fried meals, dense carbs that put you to sleep and high-sodium foods that bloat you to the point of discomfort.

Thousands of books have been written about healthy eating, and it would be easy to reinvent the wheel here and cover the same familiar ground. Instead, we will take a more cholesterol-focused approach and present two specific eating plans that have shown to be helpful in combating unhealthy cholesterol levels.

First, we'll look at the government-sanctioned Therapeutic Lifestyle Change (TLC) program, designed by the National Cholesterol Educational Program (NCEP) of the National Heart, Lung, and Blood Institute (NHLBI) of the National Institutes of Health (NIH). How's that for a mouthful! From here on, we'll forget the bureaucratic labels and refer to it as the TLC program.

Then, because we believe that it's always easier to succeed when you have choices, we will present the popular Mediterranean Diet. The two eating plans take somewhat different approaches to meals, so we expect that TLC may appeal to some, and the Mediterranean Diet to others. Also, we've modified TLC slightly to update it; our version emphasizes more whole foods and fewer refined, "simple" carbohydrates than the original. And throughout the chapter, we will provide tips on how to incorporate some of your favorite foods into your new, healthy food plan.

At the end of the chapter, we've provided a nutrition counter with the nutrient content of foods commonly found in American kitchens. Most of these are "whole foods" rather than processed; you can read the labels on the packages to learn about the nutrients in processed items. In Chapter 6, we'll talk about making healthy choices in life situations, including dining out; at the end of that chapter we will provide a nutrition counter for foods served in popular chain restaurants.

GIVE YOUR HEART SOME TLC!

The TLC program is more than a plan for lowering your cholesterol with heart-healthy foods, though that's certainly its primary mission. TLC actually is a step-by-step program for achieving an overall healthy lifestyle—TLC, remember, stands for Therapeutic Lifestyle Changes—and includes such other lifestyle factors as exercise, weight loss and medication if necessary, all working together to reduce your LDL cholesterol levels and your risk of developing heart disease. We will cover the other lifestyle aspects of the TLC program in later chapters that address exercise, relaxation and other lifestyle changes.

If your cholesterol levels are too high, this is the plan developed by the NIH and recommended by many hospitals and physicians. If you also carry excess pounds, you already know that weight loss will be one of your most important goals in creating a heart-healthy lifestyle; this, too, is a central part of TLC for those who need to trim down.

Here's the TLC program in a nutshell.

TLC happens in three stages. The first step of each stage is a visit to your physician. In Phase I, you begin your new lifestyle by eating fewer saturated fats and trans fats and less cholesterol, and by gradually increasing your physical activity. If you carry excess weight, you also begin eating fewer calories and, to help make that happen, you start incorporating more fiber into your diet so that you will become fuller without eating so many calories as before. This phase continues for six weeks.

Phase II of TLC starts with your second doctor's visit, so that you can measure the improvements your lifestyle changes already have made to your LDL! With this phase you begin gradually increasing your intake of soluble fiber, and you add plant stanols and sterols to your diet. Stanols and sterols (or "phytosterols"), you remember, are natural compounds found in the membranes of plant cells. They block absorption of dietary cholesterol because they structurally resemble the cholesterol produced by your body, so adding them to your diet can make a big difference in reducing your LDL levels—as much as 14 percent in one study. You and your doctor also discuss your diet during this visit, and make any necessary adjustments. Your physical activity should be gradually increasing. Phase II lasts for another six weeks.

Phase III of TLC is a milestone. You've been on the program for 12 weeks, and if your lifestyle changes haven't brought about the reductions to your LDL that you anticipated, you may want to discuss drug therapy to get your LDL reduced. You will also continue discussing your weight loss, physical activity and diet challenges. After this visit, you will continue following the TLC regimens custom-designed by you and your doctor, and schedule follow-up visits every four to six months.

CALORIES: THE CORNERSTONE OF ANY DIET PLAN

You've heard it before: calories in, calories out. The most reliable and safe way to lose weight is to spend or burn more calories than you eat. We'll talk about exercise and burning calories in Chapter 8, but first you need to decide: what will your calorie limit be?

This is an important decision, and it should be part of your initial talk with your doctor as you begin the TLC plan. It's difficult to generalize because everyone's weight goals, metabolic rates, exercise levels, weight loss rates and food preferences are different—but the rule of thumb is, women and men trying to lose weight should eat between 1,200 and 1,800 calories per day.

WHAT'S A SERVING?

So, you think you know portion control? Take the interactive TLC quiz at http://hin.nhlbi.nih.gov/portion to see how close your guesses come to "official" portion sizes. Here's a cheat sheet for your reference.

1 Serving of Grains

1 cup of cereal flakes = a fist
1 pancake = a compact disc
½ cup of cooked rice, pasta, or potato = ½ baseball
1 slice of bread = a cassette tape
1 piece of cornbread = a bar of soap

1 Serving of Fruits and Vegetables

1 medium fruit = a baseball
½ cup of fresh fruit = ½ baseball
¼ cup of raisins = a large egg
1 cup of salad greens = a baseball
1 baked potato = a fist

1 Serving of Milk

1½ oz cheese = 4 stacked dice or 2 cheese slices
½ cup ice cream = ½ baseball

1 Serving of Fats or Oils

1 tsp margarine or spreads = 1 die

1 Serving of Lean Meat and Beans

3 oz meat, fish and poultry = a deck of cards
3 oz grilled/baked fish = a checkbook
2 tbsp peanut butter = a Ping-Pong ball

THE TLC DIET: AN OVERVIEW

Here's where you will see that the TLC diet is anything but a starvation diet! Many people, even those who normally eat hearty meals, find it difficult to take in all of the servings listed on this diet. All you need to do in order to succeed is to make sure each serving is a heart-healthy choice.

Breads/Cereals/Grains: Six or more servings a day, as long as they fit into your calorie limits and are made of complex carbohydrates—low in saturated fat, cholesterol and total fat. These include whole-grain breads and cereals, whole wheat pasta, brown rice, and low-fat whole-grain crackers.

Vegetables: Three to five servings a day. Here is where you will find much of your day's quota of vitamins, fiber and other important nutrients. Peas also are great sources of plant protein. You can buy these fresh, frozen or canned, as long as they have no added fat, sauce or salt.

Fruits: Two to four servings a day. These, too, will give you plenty of vitamins, fiber and other nutrients. Fresh, frozen, canned or dried are all acceptable, as long as they have no added sugar.

Dairy Products: Two to three servings a day, fat-free or low-fat (example: 1% milk). Low- and no-fat dairy products provide as much or more calcium and protein as whole-milk dairy products, but without the saturated fat. Fat-free or low-fat milk, buttermilk, yogurt, sour cream, cream cheese, low-fat cheese all qualify. The cutoff is 3 grams of fat per ounce.

Eggs: Two or fewer yolks per week, including yolks in baked goods, and in cooked or processed foods. People with healthy cholesterol levels can eat up to six egg yolks per week without concern, but the yolks are high in cholesterol; if your levels are even moderately high it's best to cut back on the yolks. Instead, use egg substitutes, which contain no dietary cholesterol and far fewer calories than whole eggs.

Meat/Poultry/Fish: Five or ounces less a day. To keep the saturated fat low, eat poultry without the skin, fish, and lean cuts of meat. Remove fat or skin before cooking. For lean cuts of beef, try sirloin tip, round steak, rump roast, extra-lean hamburger and cold cuts made with lean meat. For lean pork, look for loin chops and pork tenderloin. Organ meats such as brain, liver and kidneys are high in cholesterol, so limit those items in your diet. Surprisingly, even though shrimp is very low-calorie, it's high in cholesterol, so eat it sparingly.

Fats/Oils: Keep your calories in mind when eating all fats and oils. Nuts are high in fat and calories, so eat them in moderation. For vegetable oils that contain healthier fats, try canola, corn, olive, safflower and soybean oils. Soft or liquid margarines are better than stick margarine, which is high in saturated fat. (Remember: If the label says the oil is hydrogenated or partially hydrogenated, it's high in saturated fat.) The number to remember: One gram of saturated fat per serving means the food can be labeled "low" in saturated fat.

Soluble Fiber: Choose barley, oats, psyllium, apples, bananas, berries, citrus fruits, nectarines, peaches, pears, plums, prunes, broccoli, Brussels sprouts, carrots, dry beans, peas, and soy products such as tofu and miso.

OATMEAL, THE CHAMPION OF LOWER CHOLESTEROL

If you reach for a dish of oatmeal every morning, your arteries and heart will be most grateful.

Not only has oatmeal been proven to lower LDL levels, it also helps your endothelial function—that is, your arteries' ability to dilate continually and keep your blood flowing to your heart and throughout your body.

When a person is overweight or develops metabolic syndrome, the endothelial function is, in a word, dysfunctional. The arteries don't dilate well and the blood flow is sluggish. But a study reported in the *Journal of the American College of Nutrition* found that by eating a daily bowl of oatmeal for just six weeks, the participants' endothelium—the lining of the blood vessels—functioned well once again.

To boost the nutrients in your morning oatmeal even more, sprinkle it with a handful of fresh or frozen blueberries and a tablespoon of sliced, toasted, unsalted almonds.

SNACKING ON THE TLC PROGRAM

Contrary to what most of us were taught, it *is* possible—even advisable—to snack and lose weight. You just need to be mindful of your daily calorie limits and the nutrients we've already discussed; a 150-calorie apple will be far healthier, and do more for your weight-loss goals, than 150 calories' worth of salty potato chips or a chocolate-covered donut!

TLC guidelines list the following as between-meal snacks that shouldn't deter you from your weight loss or heart-healthy goals. As mentioned earlier, we've modified some food selections to give you healthier choices.

Snacks

- Fresh or frozen fruits
- Fresh vegetables such as blanched asparagus spears, bell pepper strips, celery or carrots
- Popped corn (best air popped, without added butter or salt)
- Low-fat or fat-free whole-grain or whole-wheat crackers
- Melba toast
- Low-fat string cheese
- Whole-grain bagel
- Whole-grain English muffin
- Ready-to-eat cereals made with whole grains

Sweets

- Fresh fruits
- Low-fat or fat-free fruit yogurt
- Frozen low-fat or fat-free yogurt
- Fruit ices, no added sugar
- Sherbet
- Sugar-free Jell-O

TIPS FOR COOKING HEART-HEALTHY MEALS
THAT TASTE GREAT

As you start assembling your heart-healthy meals following TLC guidelines, use these tips to make them as tasty as those artery-clogging foods you ate in your former life. I dare you to notice the difference!

Cooking

- Set aside the butter and high-fat sauces. Use reduced-sodium vegetable broth, vegetables, small amounts of vegetable oil or cooking spray.

- Instead of frying, switch to baking, broiling, roasting, steaming, poaching, lightly stir-frying, microwaving or sautéing.

- When you're finished cooking a soup or stew, refrigerate it for a few hours. Then take it out of the refrigerator and skim the fat off the top.

- Use spices and herbs when you prepare stews, soups and other dishes, and very little salt.

Milk/Cream/Sour Cream

- Instead of sour cream, blend 1 cup low-fat, unsalted cottage cheese with 1 tablespoon fat-free milk and 2 tablespoons lemon juice, or substitute fat-free or low-fat sour cream or yogurt.

- To make dips, use flavorful Greek yogurt instead of high-fat mayonnaise or sour cream.

- Cook with low-fat or fat-free milk instead of whole milk or cream.

Spices/Flavorings

- Always buy low-sodium bouillons and broth.

- Instead of bacon, use a small amount of skinless smoked turkey breast to flavor dishes.

- Use skinless chicken thighs instead of neck bones in soups and other dishes.

Oils/Butter

- Read the labels! Buy margarine that lists liquid vegetable oil as the first ingredient, and is free of trans fat and low in saturated fat.

- Diet margarines often don't work in baking. Use regular soft margarine made with vegetable oil. Don't use lard, butter or other fats that are hard at room temperature.

Eggs

- When you bake or cook, use three egg whites and just one egg yolk instead of two whole eggs—or two egg whites or ¼ cup of egg substitute instead of one whole egg.

Sandwiches/Salads

- Use fat-free or low-fat dressing, yogurt or mayonnaise.

- To make a tasty salad dressing, use equal parts water and vinegar, and half as much oil as usual.

- Garnish green salads with fruits and vegetables to fill you up.

Breads

- When you bake muffins, breads and biscuits, use no more than 1-2 tablespoons of fat for each cup of flour.

- Substitute three ripe, very well mashed bananas for ½ cup butter or oil. Or, substitute a cup of applesauce for a cup of butter, margarine, oil or shortening, for less saturated fat and far fewer calories.

Desserts

- Don't think in terms of denying yourself dessert—think of ways you can make them heart-healthy.

- For chocolate desserts, use 3 tablespoons of cocoa instead of 1 ounce of baking chocolate. If the fat from the chocolate is necessary, add 1 tablespoon or less of vegetable oil.

- When you make cakes and soft-drop cookies, use no more than 2 tablespoons of fat for each cup of flour.

MAKING IT TASTIER!

Are you still a little lost because you can't salt up your foods? The TLC program offers these substitutes to make your foods taste better than ever.

With beef: marjoram, nutmeg, onion, pepper, sage, thyme.
With lamb: curry powder, garlic, rosemary, mint.
With pork: garlic, onion, sage, pepper, oregano.
With veal: bay leaf, curry powder, ginger, marjoram, oregano.
With chicken: ginger, marjoram, oregano, paprika,

poultry seasoning, rosemary, sage, tarragon, thyme.

With fish: curry powder, dill, dry mustard, lemon juice, marjoram, paprika, pepper.

With carrots: cinnamon, cloves, marjoram, nutmeg, rosemary, sage.

With corn: cumin, curry powder, onion, paprika, parsley.

With green beans: dill, curry powder, lemon juice, marjoram, oregano, tarragon, thyme.

With greens: onion, pepper.

With peas: ginger, marjoram, onion, parsley, sage.

With potatoes: dill, garlic, onion, paprika, parsley, sage.

With summer squash: cloves, curry powder, marjoram, nutmeg, rosemary, sage.

With winter squash: cinnamon, ginger, nutmet, onion.

With tomatoes: basil, bay leaf, dill, marjoram, onion, oregano, parsley, pepper.

TRICKS FOR CUTTING CALORIES

If the TLC program is anything, it's realistic—and the smart people who developed the plan know that cutting calories is a lifestyle change that takes time. They offer these suggestions for reducing calories—and they're so simple, you could do them every day for the rest of your life:

- You may think it's a cliché, but it works: Drinking water helps you to feel full. Drink eight 8-ounce glasses a day and you won't reach for food so often.

- Keep fresh or steamed vegetables cleaned, cut and handy for when you feel a bit hungry between meals.

- Start meals with a cup of low-calorie, low-fat broth-based soup.

- You need protein to build muscle as you lose weight, but it doesn't have to add fat to your diet. An ounce of fat-free or low-fat cheese will help. Try reduced-fat string cheese, available at any supermarket—each piece is packed with 9 grams of protein!

- Cut back your red-meat intake (beef, veal, lamb or pork) to just once or twice a week.

- Most fruits have less than 100 calories per serving, and they're dense with fiber, antioxidants and other valuable nutrients. Half a mango or grapefruit, a cup of melon cubes or berries, or a fresh kiwi or orange can be a satisfying mid-day treat.

- Always buy reduced-calorie, whole-grain bread; you'll get both flavor and fiber, and most types are just 40 calories a slice.

- Look for ways to cut calories as you cook and eat. Use salsa instead of butter for topping potatoes; bake "French fries" tossed in olive oil and herbs; substitute yams for white potatoes.

GETTING MORE FIBER

In the nutrition counter at the end of this chapter, you will see fiber counts for the most common foods we use at home. TLC recommends that, in order to lower your LDL cholesterol levels, you get at least 5 to 10 grams of soluble fiber a day—and, preferably, up to 25 grams to lower your LDL levels even more.

However, don't try to boost your fiber intake all at once. Add whole grains gradually, perhaps with oatmeal or a whole-grain cold cereal in the morning, for the first couple of weeks. A sudden increase in fiber can cause cramping and bloating. After a few days of eating higher-fiber cereal, add berries, a banana or apple to your cereal for more fiber.

If you don't have high-fiber cereal, add a few spoonfuls of unprocessed wheat bran to whatever cereal you're eating, or stir cooked barley into your scrambled eggs.

Always reach for the whole fruit, if you can, rather than fruit juice. An orange, for instance, provides *six* times more fiber than one 4-ounce glass of orange juice.

Another fiber-boosting tip: Add black beans to your salads. They're compatible with any salad type or flavor of dressing, and they add good fiber.

HOW MUCH FAT IS TOO MUCH?

If you have unhealthy cholesterol levels or are trying to lose weight, the TLC program offers guidelines for the amount of fat you should eat every day: Your total fat intake can be up to 25 to 35 percent of your daily calories. Sound generous? That's because they want you to have enough flexibility in your food that you'll stick with TLC for life.

Your saturated fat intake, however, should be no more than 7 percent of your calories every day. Here's a quick reference guide to help you follow that advice:

If you consume: Calories/day	Eat no more than: Saturated fat*
1,200	8 g
1,500	10 g
1,800	12 g
2,000	13 g
2,500	17 g

You can see how easily you can track your fat intake. Once you decide on your daily calorie goal, and become accustomed to looking at the calorie counts in foods you

---

* Fat measures shown equal about 6 percent of total calories.

like to eat, it will be easy to then plan your fat quota for the day.

WHAT GOOD WILL THIS TLC DO?

You're wondering whether following the TLC program is worth it. The answer, according to thousands of people who tested it, is absolutely, scientifically, Yes!

Here are the changes in your LDL levels that you can realistically expect to see if you follow the TLC program.

	Change	LDL Reduction
Saturated fat	Decrease to less than 7% of calories ingested	8–10%
Dietary cholesterol	Decrease to less than 200 mg/day	3–5%
Weight	Lose 10 lbs if overweight	5–8%
Soluble fiber	Add 5–10 g/day	3–5%
Plant sterols/ stanols	Add 2 g/day	5–15%
Total LDL reduction		20–30%

THE MEDITERRANEAN DIET

The Mediterranean diet wasn't invented; it evolved. Researchers in the mid-twentieth century noticed that people living in some Mediterranean regions not only enjoyed an extraordinarily long life expectancy, they also had some of the lowest heart disease, cancer, and other diet-related rates in the world. The American Heart Association (AHA) cites these dietary factors worth noting for heart health:

- People in Mediterranean regions eat far more plant foods than Americans.

- The Mediterranean diet is primarily a whole-foods diet, more so than even the TLC program, and discourages eating processed foods.

- The Mediterranean diet allows for more fats than most other weight-loss plans, which might appeal to some individuals. (Healthy fats only—no trans fats!) It also allows more fats than the standard AHA recommendations. But because it doesn't allow for processed foods, the Mediterranean diet also involves more cooking.

- Olive oil is the main source of fat in the Mediterranean diet. As you recall from Chapter 4, olive oil is a better choice because it's a monounsaturated fatty acid, or MUFA—a healthy fat that helps lower your LDL cholesterol and, consequently, your risk of coronary heart disease.

- People following the diet eat fish and poultry in moderate amounts, and just a small amount of red meat.

- Dairy products, too, are eaten in moderation, mostly cheese and yogurt.

- Eggs are on the diet, but in moderate amounts (two to four per week), and a moderate amount of wine (one to two glasses per day, usually with meals).

• Dessert is typically fresh fruit; sweets are rarely eaten and are made with honey.

Physical activity is important to the Mediterranean diet plan—not surprising, since the regions surrounding the Mediterranean are hilly. Considering all of these factors, the International Task Force for Prevention of Coronary Heart Disease concluded that the Mediterranean diet may reduce the risk of atherosclerosis and coronary heart disease, largely because people who followed it ate a reduced amount of saturated fatty acids; they substituted monounsaturated fatty acids and oils, plus ate more vegetables, fruit and whole grains than their counterparts in other regions around the world.

They found that LDL cholesterol and triglycerides were reduced by following the Mediterranean diet, HDL was elevated and metabolic syndrome was diminished—all because they ate a diet of whole foods, and little or no processed foods.

What's more, the Lyon Heart Study, published in *Circulation: Journal of the American Heart Association* several years later, found that people who followed a Mediterranean diet after experiencing a heart attack were 50 percent to 70 percent less likely to have a second heart attack than people who followed a "Western" diet.

COUNTING NUTRIENTS FOR HEALTHY CHOLESTEROL

By now you understand the impact your foods can have on your cholesterol levels—and, consequently, on your heart health. This nutrition counter will deepen your understanding of the various nutrients in your foods and make it easier to plan your meals every day. You can use the counter to take your heart-health expertise to the next level: You prepare meals with a much fuller knowledge of the food you'll be eating and serving to your family!

As you plan a meal, keep portion size in mind; the sizes

in our counter reflect standards used by the U.S. Department of Agriculture (USDA) and food manufacturers. Yes, we all know that half a cup of ice cream isn't a real serving in anyone's home—but if you serve more than that amount, you're adding calories, fat and other nutrients. And you can always "doctor up" a single scoop with unsalted nuts, bananas or unsweetened dried fruit, and a dollop of real whipped cream to transform it into a gourmet treat.

The measures here—calories, fat, saturated fat, sodium, carbohydrates, fiber and sugar—have been included because they all influence weight loss (which, you remember, is the single most important lifestyle factor in reaching healthy cholesterol levels), and in some instances, they directly impact your cholesterol. You've read about these components in earlier chapters, but here is a quick recap for your reference.

- *Calories,* in technical terms, tell you the amount of energy in one serving of any food. What makes them meaningful to you is that, in order to lose weight, you must "burn" more calories than you consume. For long-term weight loss at a healthy pace, most experts agree that between 1,200 and 1,500 per day will give most people the fuel they need for the day.

- *Fats* can be confusing. The total fat amount in this counter includes all fats in the food; you want to look for products with more *polyunsaturated* fats, especially Omega-3 fatty acids, the healthier fats found in plant foods such as nuts and healthy oils, and in cold water fish, such as salmon.

- *Saturated fat,* as you read in Chapter 4, is the subject of much ongoing research. Scientists still agree, though, that an excess of saturated fat—the kinds of fat that are solid at room temperature, such as butter, lard, and fatty meats—boosts your risk of cardiovascular disease. Saturated fats should account for less than 10 percent of your daily calories, or the equivalent of less than two pats of butter.

• Your best bet is to read labels as you shop, a topic we'll cover more thoroughly in Chapter 6, and look for the word "hydrogenated"—a clear indicator that the food contains trans fats—the worst fats of all.

• *Sodium*'s biggest danger is its ability to increase blood pressure, thereby increasing your heart disease risk. People who have not been diagnosed with blood pressure problems should take in no more than 1,500 milligrams of sodium per day, according to the National Heart, Lung, and Blood Institute. That's about 1 teaspoon of salt. Your salt intake will be easier to control, of course, if you rely more on fresh foods rather than frozen, canned or processed, which can be extremely high in sodium content.

• *Carbohydrates* can contribute to high cholesterol levels. Carbs are processed by the body, converting to blood glucose—essential to our daily energy. Too much blood glucose, however, becomes triglycerides, the type of blood fat we discussed so much in earlier chapters. We store them in our fatty tissues, gain weight, and often increase our LDL. We need carbohydrates; those from whole grains, fruits and vegetables give us energy, but those in white flour, white potatoes and sweets bring fewer nutrients into our systems and should be a small part of your daily eating plan, especially if you're trying to lose weight.

• *Fiber* is the master of weight control because it makes us feel full without added calories. It helps us digest our food and keeps us "regular," and soluble fiber—found in oats, seeds (including flax), carrots, soy, wheat bran and bananas—helps to lower our

LDL cholesterol. The optimal daily count is 25 to 30 grams of fiber per day, including at least 5 to 10 grams of soluble fiber.

• *Sugar,* as mentioned above, converts to glucose in our bodies and packs on the pounds—not to mention contributing to high blood sugar, insulin resistance and, ultimately, a higher risk of heart disease.

The amounts shown here are for foods commonly found in the kitchen and used in cooking at home. At the end of Chapter 6—the chapter where we'll discuss making sound choices in real-life situations, such as dining out—you will find a much lengthier nutrient counter containing nutritional information on menu items at popular restaurants.

Foods are listed alphabetically within categories such as breads, dairy, and nuts. Where you see the abbreviation "na" instead of a number, it means that piece of information was not available. Other abbreviations:

• tbsp = tablespoon
• tsp = teaspoon
• ea = each
• g = grams
• lg = large
• med = medium
• sm = small
• oz = ounce
• pc = piece
• reg = regular
• w/ = with
• w/o = without

The above abbreviations apply to the nutrient counter following Chapter 6 as well; that counter gives nutrition amounts for foods served in popular restaurants. Note, too, that amounts of various nutrients are given in their standard formats.

Fats and Saturated Fats (SatFat) amounts are shown
   in grams (g);
Sodium is in milligrams (mg);
Carbohydrates are in grams (g);
Fiber is in grams;
Sugar is in grams.

Information was gathered from U.S. government data, the
USDA National Nutrient Database, and a number of print
and Internet sources, including MayoClinic.com, FoodCount
.com, PennMedicine.org, and AAKP.org.

NUTRITION COUNTER FOR PREPARING FOOD AT HOME

Beans, Nuts & Seeds	Cals	Fat (g)	SatFat (g)
Almonds, 1 cup	529	45	3
Almonds, dry roasted w/o salt, 1 cup	824	73	6
Almonds, oil roasted w/o salt, 1 cup	953	87	7
Almond paste, 1 oz.	130	8	1
Black beans, cooked, boiled w/o salt, 1 cup	227	1	0
Brazil nuts, 1 cup	872	88	20
Cashews, dry roasted, w/o salt, 1 cup	786	64	13
Cashews, oil roasted, w/o salt, 1 cup	748	62	11
Chestnuts, boiled & steamed, 1 oz	43	0	0
Chickpeas, canned, 1 cup	286	3	0
Coconut meat, raw, 1 cup	283	27	24
Coconut meat, dried, unsweetened, 1 cup	187	18	16
Coconut cream, raw, 1 tbsp	50	5	5
Filberts or hazelnuts, blanched, 1 oz	178	17	1
Kidney beans, cooked, w/o salt, 1 cup	225	1	0
Lentils, cooked, boiled, w/o salt, 1 cup	230	1	0
Lima beans, lg, cooked, boiled, w/o salt, 1 cup	216	1	0
Macadamia nuts, raw, 1 oz	204	21	3

Sodium (mg)	Carbs (g)	Fiber (g)	Sugar (g)
1	20	11	4
1	27	16	7
2	28	17	7
3	14	1	10
2	41	15	na
4	16	10	3
22	45	4	7
17	39	4	6
1	10	na	na
718	54	11	na
16	12	7	5
10	7	5	2
1	1	0	na
0	5	3	1
2	40	11	1
4	40	16	4
4	39	13	5
1	4	2	1

Beans, Nuts & Seeds	Cals	Fat (g)	SatFat (g)
Macadamia nuts, oil roasted w/o salt, 1 cup	962	103	15
Peanuts, dry roasted w/salt, 1 oz	166	14	2
Pecans, dry roasted w/o salt, 1 oz	201	21	1
Pecans, oil roasted w/o salt, 1 oz	203	21	2
Pine nuts, dry roasted w/o salt, 1 cup	702	57	7
Soybeans, cooked, w/o salt, 1 cup	298	15	2

Peanut & Soy Products

	Cals	Fat (g)	SatFat (g)
Peanut butter, chunky, 2 tbsp	188	16	3
Peanut butter, smooth, 2 tbsp	188	16	4
Soy milk, 1 cup	131	4	1
Soy sauce, 1 tbsp	11	0	0
Tempeh, 1 cup	320	18	4
Tofu, raw, reg, 1 cup	151	9	1

Breads, Grains & Pasta

BREADS
	Cals	Fat (g)	SatFat (g)
Bagel, plain, 1	146	1	0
Bagel, cinnamon-raisin, 1	156	1	0
Bagel, oat bran, 1	145	1	0
Bread crumbs, dry, plain, 1 cup	427	6	1

Sodium (mg)	Carbs (g)	Fiber (g)	Sugar (g)
9	17	12	na
230	6	2	1
0	4	3	1
0	4	3	1
12	34	13	10
2	17	10	5
156	7	3	3
147	6	2	3
124	15	2	10
1005	1	0	0
15	16	na	na
20	4	1	2
255	29	1	3
184	31	1	3
289	30	2	1
791	78	5	7

Breads, Grains & Pasta	Cals	Fat (g)	SatFat (g)
BREADS			
Breadsticks, plain, 1 small	21	0	0
Dinner roll, wheat, 1 roll, 1 oz	76	2	0
English muffin, plain, 1	129	1	0
English muffin, whole-wheat, 1	134	1	0
Hamburger or hot dog bun, 1	120	2	0
Italian bread, 1 slice	81	1	0
Mixed-grain bread, 1 slice	109	2	0
Oatmeal bread, 1 slice	73	1	0
Phyllo dough, 1 sheet	57	1	0
Pita, white, enriched bread, 1	165	1	0
Pita, whole-wheat bread, 1	170	2	0
Raisin, enriched bread, 1 slice	88	1	0
Rye bread, 1 slice	83	1	0
Wheat or wheat berry bread, 1 slice	66	1	0
Tortilla, corn, 1	52	1	0
Tortilla, flour, 1	94	1	9
Oyster crackers, 1 cup	189	4	1
Wheat crackers, 1 pc	9	0	0
FLOUR, 1 CUP			
Buckwheat, whole-groat	402	4	1
Cornmeal, whole-grain, white	442	4	1

Sodium (mg)	Carbs (g)	Fiber (g)	Sugar (g)
33	3	0	0
95	13	1	0
242	25	2	2
312	27	4	5
206	21	1	3
175	15	1	0
172	18	3	3
162	13	1	2
92	10	0	0
322	33	1	1
340	35	5	1
125	17	1	2
211	15	2	1
130	12	1	1
11	10	2	1
191	15	1	1
502	33	1	1
16	1	0	0
13	85	12	3
43	94	9	1

Breads, Grains & Pasta	Cals	Fat (g)	SatFat (g)
FLOUR, 1 CUP			
Cornmeal, whole-grain, yellow	440	2	0
Wheat flour, whole-grain	651	5	0
Wheat flour, white, all-purpose, enriched	455	1	0
GRAINS, 1 CUP			
Barley, pearled, cooked	193	1	0
Corn grits, white, reg or quick, enriched cooked w/water, salt	143	0	0
Corn grits, yellow, reg or quick, enriched cooked w/water, w/o salt	143	0	0
Couscous, cooked	176	0	0
Farina, unenriched, dry	649	1	0
Hominy, canned, white	119	1	0
Hominy, canned, yellow	115	1	0
Oat bran, cooked	88	2	0
Oats, reg, quick or instant, cooked w/water, w/o salt	166	3	1
Quinoa, cooked	222	4	na
Rice, brown, long-grain, cooked	216	2	0
Rice, brown, medium-grain, cooked	218	2	0
Rice, white, long-grain, reg, cooked, enriched, w/salt	205	0	0
Semolina, enriched	601	2	0

Sodium (mg)	Carbs (g)	Fiber (g)	Sugar (g)
32	93	3	0
4	137	na	na
2	95	3	0
5	44	6	0
140	31	0	0
5	31	0	0
8	36	2	0
5	137	3	na
346	24	4	3
336	23	4	na
2	25	6	na
9	28	4	1
13	39	5	na
10	45	4	1
2	46	4	na
604	45	1	0
2	122	7	na

Breads, Grains & Pasta	Cals	Fat (g)	SatFat (g)
GRAINS, 1 CUP			
Sorghum	651	6	1
Wheat germ, toasted, plain	432	12	2
Wild rice, cooked	166	1	0
PASTA, 1 CUP			
Macaroni, cooked, enriched, elbow shape	221	1	0
Macaroni, whole-wheat, cooked elbow shape	174	1	0
Noodles, egg, cooked, enriched	221	3	1
Noodles, egg, spinach, cooked, enriched	211	3	1
Noodles, Chinese, chow mein	237	14	2
Noodles, Japanese soba, cooked	113	0	0
Spaghetti, cooked, w/o salt, enriched	221	1	0
Spaghetti, spinach, cooked	182	1	0
Spaghetti, whole-wheat, cooked	174	1	0

Dairy

	Cals	Fat (g)	SatFat (g)
BUTTER, 1 TBSP			
Butter, w/o salt	102	12	7
Butter, w/salt	102	12	7
Butter, whipped w/salt	67	8	5

Sodium (mg)	Carbs (g)	Fiber (g)	Sugar (g)
12	143	12	na
5	56	17	9
5	35	3	1
1	43	3	1
4	37	4	1
8	40	2	1
19	39	4	1
198	26	2	0
68	24	na	na
1	43	3	1
20	37	na	na
4	37	6	1
2	0	0	0
82	0	0	0
78	0	0	0

Dairy	Cals	Fat (g)	SatFat (g)
CHEESE			
Blue, 1 oz	100	8	5
Camembert, 1 wedge	114	9	6
Cheddar, 1 cup, diced	532	44	28
Colby, 1 cup, diced	520	42	27
Cottage cheese, creamed, lg curd, 1 cup	206	9	4
Cottage cheese, uncreamed, dry, lg or sm curd, 1 cup	104	0	0
Cottage cheese, 2% fat, 1 cup	194	6	2
Cottage cheese, 1% fat, 1 cup	163	2	1
Cream cheese, 1 tbsp	50	5	3
Cream cheese, fat free, 199 g	105	1	1
Feta, 1 oz	75	6	4
Goat cheese, semisoft, 1 oz	103	8	6
Goat cheese, hard, 1 oz	128	10	7
Gouda, 1 oz	101	8	5
Gruyere, 1 cup, diced	545	43	25
Monterey, 1 cup, diced	492	40	25
Mozzarella, whole milk, 1 oz	85	6	4
Mozzarella, part skim milk, 1 oz	72	5	3
Muenster, 1 cup, diced	486	40	25
Neufchatel, 1 oz	72	6	4
Parmesan, grated, 1 tbsp	22	1	1
Provolone, 1 oz	100	8	5
Queso Anejo, crumbled, 1 cup	492	40	25

Sodium (mg)	Carb (g)	Fiber (g)	Sugar (g)
395	1	0	0
320	0	0	0
820	2	0	1
797	3	0	1
764	7	0	6
478	10	0	3
746	8	0	8
918	6	0	6
47	1	0	0
702	8	0	5
316	1	0	1
146	1	0	1
98	1	0	1
232	1	0	1
444	0	0	0
708	1	0	1
178	1	0	0
131	1	0	0
829	1	0	1
95	1	0	1
76	0	0	0
248	1	0	0
1493	6	0	6

Dairy	Cals	Fat (g)	SatFat (g)
CHEESE			
Queso Asadero, diced, 1 cup	470	37	24
Queso Chihuahua, diced, 1 cup	494	39	25
Ricotta, whole milk, 1 cup	428	32	20
Ricotta, part skim milk, 1 cup	339	19	12
Romano, 1 oz	110	8	5
Roquefort, 1 oz	105	9	5
Swiss, 1 cup, diced	502	37	23
MILK			
Whole, 3.25% fat, 1 cup	146	8	5
Lowfat, 2% fat, 1 cup	122	5	3
Lowfat, 1% fat, 1 cup	102	2	2
Skim, 1 cup	83	0	0
Buttermilk, cultured, fr/skim milk, 1 cup	98	2	1
Canned, condensed, sweetened, 1 cup	982	27	17
Canned, evaporated, whole, 1 oz.	42	2	1
Canned, evaporated, skim, 1 cup	200	1	0
Dry, skim, nonfat sol., reg, 1 cup	434	1	1
Dry, whole, 1 cup	635	34	21
CREAM			
Half and half, 1 tbsp	20	2	1
Sour cream, cultured, 1 cup	444	45	30

Sodium (mg)	Carb (g)	Fiber (g)	Sugar (g)
865	4	0	4
814	7	0	7
207	7	0	1
308	13	0	1
340	1	0	0
513	1	0	na
253	7	0	2
98	11	0	13
100	11	0	12
107	12	0	13
103	12	0	12
257	12	0	12
389	166	0	166
33	3	0	na
294	29	0	29
642	62	0	62
475	49	0	49
6	1	0	0
184	7	0	8

Dairy	Cals	Fat (g)	SatFat (g)
CREAM			
Sour cream, cultured, 1 tbsp	23	2	1
Sour cream, imitation, cultured, 1 cup	478	45	41
Whipping cream, light, 1 cup, fluid (yields 2 cups whipped)	698	74	46
Whipping cream, heavy, 1 cup, fluid (yields 2 cups whipped)	821	88	55
Whipping cream, heavy, 1 tbsp	52	6	3
ICE CREAM, ½ CUP			
Ice cream, chocolate	143	7	4
Ice cream, strawberry	127	6	3
Ice cream, vanilla	137	7	4
Ice cream, vanilla, light	125	4	2
YOGURT, 1 CUP			
Plain, whole milk	149	8	5
Plain, lowfat	154	4	2
Plain, skim milk	137	0	0

Fats & Oils

FATS			
Lard, 1 tbsp	115	13	5
Margarine, reg, hard, corn, 1 tsp	34	4	1

Sodium (mg)	Carb (g)	Fiber (g)	Sugar (g)
10	0	0	0
235	15	0	15
81	7	0	0
90	7	0	0
6	0	0	0
50	19	1	17
40	18	1	na
53	16	1	14
56	20	0	17
113	11	0	11
172	17	0	17
189	19	0	19
0	0	0	0
44	0	0	0

Fats & Oils	Cals	Fat (g)	SatFat (g)
FATS			
Margarine, soft, corn, 1 tsp	34	4	1
Margarine blend, 60% corn oil, 40% butter, 1 tbsp	102	11	4
OILS, 1 TBSP			
Almond oil	120	14	1
Canola oil	124	14	1
Corn, salad or cooking oil	120	14	2
Grapeseed	120	14	1
Olive, salad or cooking oil	119	14	2
Peanut, salad or cooking oil	119	14	2
Sesame, salad or cooking oil	120	14	2
Soybean, salad or cooking oil (hydrog.)	120	14	2

Fruits

	Cals	Fat (g)	SatFat (g)
Apple, raw w/skin, 3.25"	116	0	0
Apples, dried, sulfured, uncooked, 1 cup	209	0	0
Apple juice, unsweetened, w/vit. C, 1 cup	114	0	0
Applesauce, unsweetened, 1 cup	102	0	0
Apricots, raw, 1 cup	74	1	0

Sodium (mg)	Carbs (g)	Fiber (g)	Sugar (g)
51	0	0	0
127	0	0	0
0	0	0	0
0	0	0	0
0	0	0	0
0	0	0	0
0	0	0	0
0	0	0	0
0	0	0	0
0	0	0	0
2	31	5	23
75	57	7	49
10	28	1	24
5	28	3	23
2	17	4	14

Fruits	Cals	Fat (g)	SatFat (g)
Apricots, canned, juice pk, w/skin, sol. & liquids, 1 cup, halves	117	0	0
Apricots, dried, sulfured, uncooked, 1 half	8	0	0
Apricot nectar, canned, 1 cup	141	0	0
Avocados, raw, Calif., 1 w/o skin & seeds	227	21	3
Avocados, raw, Fla., 2 w/o skin & seeds	365	31	6
Banana, raw, 1 cup, sliced	134	0	0
Blackberries, raw, 1 cup	62	1	0
Blueberries, raw, 1 cup	84	0	0
Cherries, sour, red, raw, 1 cup w/pits	52	0	0
Cherries, sweet, raw, 1 cup w/pits	87	0	0
Clementine, raw, 1 fruit	35	0	na
Cranberries, dried, sweetened, 1 cup	383	2	0
Cranberry sauce, canned, sweetened, 1 cup	418	0	0
Currants, European, black, raw, 1 cup	71	0	0
Currants, zante, dried, 1 cup	408	0	0
Dates, domestic, 1 cup, chopped	415	1	0
Figs, dried, uncooked, 1 fig	21	0	0

Sodium (mg)	Carbs (g)	Fiber (g)	Sugar (g)
10	30	4	26
0	2	0	2
8	36	2	na
11	12	9	0
6	24	17	7
2	34	4	18
1	14	8	7
1	21	4	15
3	13	2	9
0	22	3	18
1	9	1	7
4	102	7	81
80	108	3	105
2	17	na	na
12	107	10	97
3	110	12	93
1	5	1	4

Fruits	Cals	Fat (g)	SatFat (g)
Gooseberries, canned, light syrup pk, solids & liquids, 1 cup	184	1	0
Grapefruit, raw, pink & red & white, 1 cup sections w/juice	74	0	0
Grapefruit juice, white, canned, unsweet., 1 cup	94	0	0
Grapes, red or green, 1 cup, seedless	104	0	0
Grape juice, unsweet., 1 cup	152	0	0
Kiwifruit, fresh, 1 lg	56	0	0
Lemon juice, raw, 1 oz	8	0	0
Lime juice, raw, 1 oz	8	0	0
Mango, raw, 1 pc	135	1	0
Melon, cantaloupe, 1 cup, balls	60	0	0
Melon, honeydew, 1 cup, diced	61	0	0
Nectarine, 1 fruit	62	0	0
Olives, ripe, 1 lg	5	0	0
Orange, Calif., 1 fruit, 2.6" diam.	59	0	0
Orange, Fla., 1 fruit, 2.7" diam.	65	0	0
Orange juice, 1 cup	112	1	0
Tangerine, 1 med.	47	0	0
Tangerines, canned, 1 cup, juice pk	92	0	0
Papayas, cubed, 1 cup	55	0	0
Passion fruit, purple, 1 fruit	17	0	0
Peach, 1 lg	68	0	0

Sodium (mg)	Carbs (g)	Fiber (g)	Sugar (g)
5	47	6	na
0	19	3	16
2	22	0	22
3	27	1	23
13	37	1	36
3	13	3	8
0	3	0	1
1	3	0	1
4	35	4	31
28	14	2	14
31	15	1	14
0	15	2	11
38	0	0	0
0	14	3	na
0	16	3	13
2	26	1	21
2	12	2	9
12	24	2	22
4	14	3	8
5	4	2	2
0	17	3	15

Fruits	Cals	Fat (g)	SatFat (g)
Peaches, dried, sulfured, 1 half	31	0	0
Pear, 1 med	103	0	0
Pineapple, raw, chunks, 1 cup	82	0	0
Pineapple juice, canned, 1 cup, unsweetened	132	0	0
Plantains, cooked, 1 cup, slices	179	0	0
Plum, 1 fruit	30	0	0
Pomegranate, raw, 1 pc	234	3	0
Pomegranate juice, 1 cup, bottled	134	1	0
Raisins, seedless, 1 cup	493	1	0
Raspberries, 1 cup	64	1	0
Rhubarb, frozen, diced, 1 cup, uncooked	29	0	0
Strawberries, halves, 1 cup, raw	49	0	0
Watermelon, balls, 1 cup	46	0	0

Herbs, Spices, Condiments

	Cals	Fat (g)	SatFat (g)
Allspice, ground, 1 tsp	5	0	0
Basil, ground, 1 tsp	7	0	0
Catsup, 1 tbsp	15	0	0
Horseradish, prepared, 1 tsp	2	0	0
Mustard, yellow, 1 tsp	3	0	0

Sodium (mg)	Carbs (g)	Fiber (g)	Sugar (g)
1	8	1	5
2	28	6	17
2	22	2	16
5	32	1	25
8	48	4	22
0	8	1	7
8	53	11	39
22	33	0	32
18	131	6	98
1	15	8	5
3	7	3	2
2	12	3	7
2	12	1	10
1	1	0	na
0	1	0	na
167	4	0	3
16	1	0	0
57	0	0	0

Herbs, Spices, Condiments	Cals	Fat (g)	SatFat (g)
Pickles, cucumber, dill, 1 cup (abt. 23 slices)	19	0	0
Pickle, cucumber, sweet, 1 cup	139	1	0
Pickle, cucumber, sour, 1 lg (4" long)	15	0	0
Pickle relish, sweet, 1 tbsp	20	0	0
Pimento, canned, 1 tbsp	3	0	0
Vanilla extract, 1 tbsp	37	0	0
Vinegar, balsamic, 1 tbsp	14	0	0
Vinegar, distilled, 1 tbsp	3	0	0
EGGS			
Whole, raw, 1 extra lg	80	6	2
Whites, raw, 1 lg	16	0	0
Yolk, raw, 1 lg	54	5	2

Meats

	Cals	Fat (g)	SatFat (g)
BEEF, 3 OZ			
Brisket	575	22	9
Chuck roast	257	16	6
Rib, roasted	298	24	10
Shortribs	400	36	15
Tenderloin	223	14	6
Ground, 95% lean	145	6	3
Ground, 70% lean	191	13	5
Ground, reg	251	19	7
Corned beef brisket	213	16	5
LAMB, 3 OZ			
Leg	162	7	2
Leg & shoulder, cubed	190	7	3

Sodium (mg)	Carbs (g)	Fiber (g)	Sugar (g)
1356	4	2	2
699	32	2	28
1631	3	2	1
122	5	0	4
2	1	0	0
1	2	0	2
4	3	na	2
0	0	0	0
78	0	0	0
55	0	0	0
8	1	0	0
146	0	0	0
42	0	0	0
54	0	0	na
42	0	0	0
48	0	0	0
55	0	0	0
57	0	0	0
65	0	0	0
964	0	0	0
58	0	0	0
60	0	0	0

Meats	Cals	Fat (g)	SatFat (g)
VEAL, 3 OZ			
Leg	128	3	1
Rib	150	6	2
Ground	146	6	3
PORK, 3 OZ			
Ham	179	8	3
Ham, cured	151	8	3
Loin	178	8	3
Center loin chops, bone-in	153	6	2
Sirloin roast, bone-in	173	8	2
Shoulder	194	11	4
Spareribs	337	26	9
BACON			
Bacon, cured, 1 slice	43	3	1
Canadian-style, 2 slices	87	4	1
CHICKEN, ½, BONELESS			
Light meat, fried, w/skin, batter	521	29	8
Light meat, fried, w/skin, flour	320	16	4
Light meat, roasted, w/skin	293	14	4
Dark meat, fried, w/skin, batter	828	52	14
Dark meat, roasted, w/skin	423	26	7
DUCK			
Meat w/skin, roasted, 1 cup	472	40	14
Meat only, roasted, 1 cup	281	16	6

Sodium (mg)	Carbs (g)	Fiber (g)	Sugar (g)
58	0	0	0
82	0	0	0
71	0	0	0
54	0	0	0
1275	0	0	0
49	0	0	0
48	0	0	0
50	0	0	0
68	0	0	na
79	0	0	0
185	0	0	0
727	1	0	0
540	18	0	na
100	2	0	0
99	0	0	na
820	26	0	na
145	0	0	na
83	0	0	0
91	0	0	0

Meats	Cals	Fat (g)	SatFat (g)
TURKEY			
Breast, w/skin, roasted, ½ breast	1633	64	18
Leg, meat, w/skin, 1 leg, roasted	1136	54	17
LUNCHEON MEAT			
Bologna, beef, 1 slice	87	8	3
Bologna, turkey, 1 serving	59	4	1
Chicken roll, light meat, 2 slices	63	2	0
Frankfurter, beef, 1	148	13	5
Frankfurter, chicken, 1	100	7	2
Frankfurter, turkey, 1	100	8	2
Ham, sliced, extra lean, 1 slice	26	1	0
Ham, sliced, reg, 1 slice	46	2	1
Salami, beef & pork, 1 slice	41	3	1
Salami, turkey, 1 servg	47	3	1
Salami, pork, 1 slice	41	3	1
Turkey breast, 1 slice	22	0	0

Seafood

	Cals	Fat (g)	SatFat (g)
FISH, COOKED			
Bass, freshwater, 3 oz	124	4	1
Bass, striped, 3 oz	105	3	1
Catfish, farmed, 3 oz	129	7	2
Caviar, black & red, 1 tbsp	40	3	1

Sodium (mg)	Carbs (g)	Fiber (g)	Sugar (g)
544	0	0	na
420	0	0	0
302	1	0	0
351	1	0	1
604	3	0	0
513	2	0	2
380	1	0	0
485	2	0	1
254	0	0	0
365	1	0	0
178	0	0	0
281	0	0	0
226	0	0	na
213	1	0	1
76	0	0	na
75	0	0	na
68	0	0	na
240	1	0	0

Seafood	Cals	Fat (g)	SatFat (g)
FISH, COOKED			
Cod, Atlantic, 3 oz	89	1	0
Eel, 1 oz, boneless	67	4	1
Grouper, 3 oz	100	1	0
Haddock, 3 oz	95	1	0
Haddock, smoked, Boneless, 1 oz	33	0	0
Halibut, Atlantic & Pacific, 3 oz	119	3	0
Monkfish, 3 oz	82	2	0
Perch, 3 oz	99	1	0
Pike, walleye, 3 oz	101	1	0
Pompano, Fla., 3 oz	179	10	4
Roughy, orange, 3 oz	89	1	0
Salmon, Chinook, reg, 3 oz, smoked (lox)	99	4	1
Salmon, Atlantic, wild, 3 oz	155	7	1
Salmon, pink, 3 oz	127	4	1
Salmon, sockeye, 3 oz	184	9	2
Sardine, Atlantic, canned in oil w/bone, 1 oz	59	3	0
Smelt, rainbow, 3 oz	105	3	0
Snapper, 3 oz	109	1	0
Swordfish, 3 oz	132	4	1
Trout, rainbow, wild, 3 oz	128	5	1
Tuna, fresh, bluefin, 3 oz	156	5	1
Tuna, fresh, yellowfin, 3 oz	118	1	0
Whitefish, smoked, 1 oz, boneless	31	0	0

Sodium (mg)	Carbs (g)	Fiber (g)	Sugar (g)
66	0	0	0
18	0	0	na
45	0	0	na
74	0	0	na
216	0	0	0
59	0	0	na
20	0	0	na
67	0	0	na
55	0	0	na
65	0	0	na
59	0	0	0
1700	0	0	na
48	0	0	na
73	0	0	na
56	0	0	na
143	0	0	0
65	0	0	na
48	0	0	na
98	0	0	na
48	0	0	na
42	0	0	na
40	0	0	na
289	0	0	0

Seafood	Cals	Fat (g)	SatFat (g)
SHELLFISH, COOKED			
Crab, Alaska king, 1 leg	130	2	0
Crab, blue, 1 cup	138	2	0
Crab, Dungeness, 1 crab	140	2	0
Crayfish, farmed, 3 oz	74	1	0
Lobster, northern, 3 oz	83	1	0
Mussel, blue, 3 oz	146	4	1
Oyster, Pacific, raw, 3 oz	69	2	0
Oyster, Pacific, moist heat, 3 oz	139	4	1
Scallops, breaded & fried, 2 large	67	3	1
Shrimp, 4 lg, moist heat	22	0	0
Squid, fried, 3 oz	149	6	2

Vegetables

	Cals	Fat (g)	SatFat (g)
Artichokes, cooked, w/o salt, 1 med	64	0	0
Arugula, raw, 1 cup	5	0	0
Asparagus, raw, small, 1 spear	2	0	0
Bamboo shoots, cooked, 1 cup w/o salt	14	0	0
Beans, snap, green, w/o salt, cooked, 1 cup	44	0	0
Beets, cooked, boiled, ½ cup slices	37	0	0
Broccoli, raw, 1 cup	31	0	0
Brussels sprouts, cooked w/o salt, ½ cup	28	0	0
Cabbage, raw, shredded, 1 cup	18	0	0

Sodium (mg)	Carbs (g)	Fiber (g)	Sugar (g)
1436	0	0	na
377	0	0	0
480	1	0	na
82	0	0	na
323	1	0	0
314	6	0	na
90	4	0	na
180	8	0	0
144	3	na	na
49	0	0	0
260	7	0	na
72	14	10	1
5	1	0	0
0	0	0	0
5	2	1	na
1	10	4	2
65	8	2	7
30	6	2	2
16	6	2	1
13	4	2	2

Vegetables	Cals	Fat (g)	SatFat (g)
Cabbage, boiled, w/o salt, ½ cup shredded	17	0	0
Carrots, raw, grated, 1 cup	45	0	0
Carrots, cooked w/o salt, ½ cup slices	27	0	0
Cauliflower, raw, 1 cup	25	0	0
Cauliflower, cooked w/o salt, ½ cup	14	0	0
Chard, Swiss, cooked w/o salt, 1 cup, chopped	35	0	0
Collards, cooked w/o salt, 1 cup, chopped	49	1	0
Corn, sweet, yellow, cooked w/o salt, 1 baby ear	9	0	0
Cucumber, w/peel, raw, ½ cup slices	8	0	0
Eggplant, cooked, w/o salt, 1 cup cubes	35	0	0
Endive, raw, chopped, ½ cup	4	0	0
Kale, cooked, chopped, 1 cup, w/o salt	36	1	0
Kohlrabi, cooked, sliced, 1 cup, w/o salt	48	0	0
Leeks, cooked, w/o salt, ¼ cup chopped	8	0	0
Lettuce, Boston or bibb, raw, 1 cup chopped	7	0	0
Lettuce, romaine, raw, ½ cup shredded	4	0	0
Lettuce, iceberg, raw, 1 cup shredded	10	0	0

Sodium (mg)	Carbs (g)	Fiber (g)	Sugar (g)
6	4	1	2
76	11	3	5
45	6	2	3
30	5	3	2
9	3	1	1
313	7	4	2
30	9	5	1
0	2	0	0
1	2	0	1
1	9	3	3
6	1	0	0
30	7	3	2
35	11	2	5
3	2	0	1
3	1	1	1
2	1	1	0
7	2	1	1

Vegetables	Cals	Fat (g)	SatFat (g)
Lettuce, looseleaf, raw, ½ cup shredded	3	0	0
Mushrooms, whole, raw, 1 cup	21	0	0
Mushrooms, shiitake, dried, 1	11	0	0
Mushrooms, shiitake, cooked w/o salt, 1 cup	81	0	0
Okra, cooked, w/o salt, 8 pods (3" long)	19	0	0
Onions, raw, chopped, 1 cup	64	0	0
Onions, cooked w/o salt, 1 cup	92	0	0
Onions, spring, raw, 1 tbsp	2	0	0
Parsley, raw, 1 cup	22	0	0
Parsnips, cooked w/o salt, ½ cup slices	55	0	0
Peas, green, cooked, w/o salt, 1 cup	134	0	0
Peppers, sweet, green, raw, chopped, 1 cup	30	0	0
Potato, baked, flesh, w/o salt, 1 potato, 2.3" × 4.75"	145	0	0
Potato skin, baked, w/o salt, 1 skin	115	0	0
Pumpkin, cooked, mashed, 1 cup w/o salt	49	0	0
Radishes, raw, slices, 1 cup	19	0	0
Spinach, cooked w/o salt, 1 cup	41	0	0

Sodium (mg)	Carbs (g)	Fiber (g)	Sugar (g)
5	1	0	0
4	3	1	2
0	3	0	0
6	21	3	5
5	4	2	2
6	15	3	7
6	21	3	10
1	0	0	0
34	4	2	1
8	13	3	4
5	25	9	9
4	7	3	4
8	34	2	3
12	27	5	1
2	12	3	3
45	4	2	2
126	7	4	1

Vegetables	Cals	Fat (g)	SatFat (g)
Squash, zucchini, raw, 1 cup, sliced incl. skin	18	0	0
Squash, acorn, cooked w/o salt, 1 cup cubes	115	0	0
Squash, butternut, cooked w/o salt, 1 cup cubes	82	0	0
Squash, spaghetti, cooked w/o salt, 1 cup	42	0	0
Sweet potato, baked in skin, w/o salt, 1 lg	162	0	0
Sweet potato, boiled, w/o skin & salt, 1 med	115	0	0
Tomatoes, red, raw, 1 cup chopped/sliced	32	0	0
Tomatoes, cooked w/o salt, 2 med	44	0	0
Turnips, cooked w/o salt, 1 cup mashed	51	0	0
Watercress, raw, chopped, 1 cup	4	0	0

Beverages

COFFEE & TEA

	Cals	Fat (g)	SatFat (g)
Coffee, brewed, 1 cup	5	0	0
Coffee, instant, 6 oz	4	0	0
Coffee, instant, decaf, 1 cup	4	0	0
Tea, brewed, 1 cup	2	0	0
Tea, herbal, chamomile, brewed, 1 cup	2	0	0

Sodium (mg)	Carbs (g)	Fiber (g)	Sugar (g)
11	4	1	2
8	30	9	na
8	22	na	4
28	10	2	4
65	37	6	12
41	27	4	9
9	7	2	5
27	10	2	6
37	12	5	7
14	0	0	0
5	1	0	0
5	1	0	0
5	1	0	0
7	1	0	0
2	0	0	0

Beverages	Cals	Fat (g)	SatFat (g)
ALCOHOLIC BEVERAGES			
Alcohol, distilled (rum, gin, vodka, whiskey), 80 proof, 1 oz	64	0	0
Alcohol, distilled (rum, gin, vodka, whiskey), 86 proof, 1 oz	70	0	0
Beer, 1 can (12 oz)	153	0	0
Beer, light, 1 can (12 oz)	103	0	0
Wine, red, 3.5 oz	74	0	0
Wine, white, 3.5 oz	70	0	0
CARBONATED BEVERAGES			
Club soda, 16 oz	0	0	0
Cola, 16 oz	202	0	0
Cola, low calorie w/aspartame, 16 oz	5	0	0
Ginger ale, 16 oz	166	0	0
Tonic water, 11 oz	114	0	0

Sodium (mg)	Carbs (g)	Fiber (g)	Sugar (g)
0	0	0	0
0	0	0	0
14	13	0	0
14	6	0	0
5	2	0	1
5	1	0	1
100	0	0	0
20	51	0	44
28	0	0	0
34	42	0	42
13	30	0	30

CHAPTER SIX

Real-Life Heart-Healthy Strategies

Knowledge, as they say, is power—and you now know which foods will help you reach healthy cholesterol goals.

But if you are like most people, you're busy. Your days are full of appointments, errands, working to keep healthy relationships, maintaining your household and probably schlepping your kids from soccer practice to ballet class to piano lesson. Who has time to track every calorie, fat gram and particle of sugar in their diets?

That's where this chapter comes in. Real life can't always be about keeping track of minute details, though it is immensely helpful to know which foods contain more saturated fats, sodium or other substances that can contribute to unhealthy cholesterol. That's why Chapter 5 included a nutrition counter, so you could begin learning to select heart-healthy foods.

This chapter, too, includes a nutrition counter—this one listing the nutrient contents of the most popular foods at restaurant chains across the country. You know you won't cook every meal at home for the rest of your life, so a quick-reference nutrition counter for a variety of restaurants will familiarize you with healthy menu choices—and teach you which ones you might want to avoid altogether (or, at least, indulge in only as a rare treat).

As you practice making healthy food choices, though, knowing the approximate nutrient counts will become almost second nature to you. While it is important to track nutrients rather precisely in the beginning, especially if you want to lose weight, you will soon learn which foods are high in sodium, for instance, and you'll steer clear. You will reach for healthy cooking oils, whole-grain breads and colorful vegetables as naturally as you once drove through your neighborhood fast-food joint.

Your food choices will become a strategy, rather than an exercise in arithmetic. You will know which foods make you feel sluggish or bloated, and you won't even *want* to eat them anymore. Your strategy, which once might have revolved around getting full by eating salty, high-fat, high-carb foods, will now aim at fueling your body to give you great energy, super concentration, fewer aches and pains, and a sunny attitude!

IT'S ALL ABOUT CHANGING YOUR BEHAVIOR

Many people with high cholesterol levels, especially if they are overweight, didn't put much thought into their food over the years.

That is, they didn't put thought into the *consequences* of their food choices. Overweight people often are fast eaters, they don't like to spend a lot of time in selecting their foods, and they are polite individuals who eat whatever they are served. If that means a giant helping of Mom's extra-cheesy lasagna, or a third piece of fried chicken, well, how much harm can one meal cause?

Eating the wrong foods can become a habit—a behavior pattern that we don't think about until after we've done it. That's the real danger in overindulging. Too often, we allow our eating to be controlled by other people—our spouses, parents, friends.

Or we eat for the wrong reasons. Most of us have reached for food when what we really crave is another half-hour of relaxation; we use food to procrastinate getting back to work or dealing with some situation we'd rather not handle.

Sometimes we eat the wrong food out of guilt, because "Mom made it especially for me," and we don't want to make the other person feel bad. We eat whatever is served at parties, and we order meals in restaurants without asking how it's prepared. All of these everyday situations are examples of giving someone *else* control over our food choices.

But they're not the ones who have to carry the extra weight, or sit up half the night with indigestion, or feel sleepy all afternoon because someone offered you pasta for lunch and you accepted. *You* are the one who has to live with the consequences of the foods you eat, so doesn't it make sense that you should be the one making the food choices?

MINDFUL EATING: ONE STRATEGY THAT WORKS

If you've heard of mindfulness, you know it is a practice that keeps us focused in this moment. What happened five minutes ago cannot be changed, and what will happen five minutes into the future can't be predicted, so the only way to truly appreciate life is to be fully aware of what's happening now.

Mindful eating is a form of mindfulness. When you eat mindfully, you set aside all other thoughts and fully experience the food you are eating—its aroma, texture and taste and how it feels going down. Mindful eating slows us down and gives our brains a chance to tell us when we are full, so that we don't *mindlessly* overeat.

It is impossible to eat mindfully if you are standing over the sink while you gulp down a sandwich, or multitasking with work at your desk. To learn mindful eating, it's best to eat alone in a quiet room; once you have mastered your mindfulness skill, you will be able to incorporate distractions into your meals, such as reading a book or dining out.

Here are the basic steps for mindful eating.

- *Focus on each bite of food.* What does it look like? What do you smell as you bring the food to your mouth? Before you start chewing, what shape is the food in your mouth? Is it too large, or very small? Cold or hot? How about its texture? If you can take the time, wait ten seconds before you start chewing each bite.

- *Put down your fork!* Don't keep your fork in your hand, poised for the next bite, and the next. Let it rest on the table between bites so you can focus on the food in your mouth—and so you'll have to pick it up again for each bite. Leave your fork on the table until you've swallowed the food in your mouth.

- *Start chewing.* How does the taste change as you chew your food? Are juices released? Your tongue has different "zones"—do you taste this bite more in the front of your tongue, where your taste buds are more attuned to sweetness, or towards the back, where they're more sensitive to bitter tastes?

- *Swallow and relax.* Have you ever noticed how your mouth and throat perform when you swallow? It's a symphony of muscles in one harmonious, almost fluid motion. As you begin swallowing each bite, notice how your tongue pushes the food back into your throat, and how your throat muscles rise to receive it.

- *Mindful eating, mindful conversation.* After you've practiced eating mindfully for a few meals, dine with your friends and family and see how easily you can incorporate the practice into social occasions. Take a bite when someone else is talking, place your fork back on the table, and absorb their viewpoint as you think about the food in your mouth. Don't reply until you've swallowed that bite, and notice how well mindful eating can transition into mindful listening!

- *Your brain thanks you.* It's not your stomach that tells you when you're full, you know—it's your brain. When you've eaten enough, nerve sensors in your stomach wall send messages to your brain, which releases neurotransmitters to tell you that you've had your fill. That doesn't happen as soon as you swallow a bite; research shows that it takes your brain about fifteen minutes to realize that you're full. So when you eat quickly and mindlessly, your brain doesn't get the message—or send it—until after you've eaten too much. Mindful eating slows it all down and gives your brain a chance to alert you that you feel full and don't want any more food. While you're eating mindfully, know that that cue is coming, and watch for it.

FOOD DIARY: ANOTHER WINNING STRATEGY

Just about every commercial diet program with a record of success—Weight Watchers, among others—recommends using the same tool to keep you aware of your goals every day: a food diary.

When you write down your food and exercise each day, you can look at your behaviors over a week's time and see your successes, along with those areas where you need to work a little harder. You will see at a glance if you tend to overeat at certain times of day. A food diary also helps you identify foods that are bringing too many calories, fat, sodium or sugar into your diet.

Have you been dipping into the peanut butter jar too often? Your food diary won't lie. Does that handful of dried cranberries add too much sugar to your breakfast cereal? Maybe you can substitute fresh or frozen, unsweetened blueberries instead.

You didn't realize you had drunk three glasses of wine on two separate occasions last week? Keeping a food diary will not only show you where you make such mistakes, but enable you to make plans for avoiding them in the future: Instead of accepting a third glass of wine, you might plan to drink a full glass of water with each alcoholic drink.

A food diary also can help you identify moods and other triggers that usually bring you to overindulge. Be a smart diarist and record what was happening each time you reached for food: Were you bored? Annoyed? Celebrating? Passing the time between meetings at work, so you grabbed some chips and a soda?

Once you identify any behavioral eating triggers, try to think of healthier replacements. If you usually reach for a midafternoon candy bar at work, give yourself a break—literally—and walk to the closest library instead. Take a few minutes to browse through their photo archives before you return to work.

Socializing with friends might be the most common eating trigger. Instead of spending the entire evening at a restaurant with food and drinks, spend two hours together at your local contemporary art museum, and finish the evening at a coffee shop discussing your favorite exhibits.

Add more fruits and vegetables to your diet—not only because they provide far better nutrients than most snack foods, but also because they're full of fiber, so they make you feel fuller without eating so many calories or fat grams. And congratulate yourself every time you ate merely because it was time for your next meal, or because you actually were hungry!

It's wise, by the way, to continue keeping your food diary even after you reach your weight loss and healthy-cholesterol goals. Experts often mention a "condition" called "calorie amnesia"—meaning, we forget to pay attention to calories and saturated fats when we select foods, and we forget to eat mindfully. As long as you record your food and exercise every day, you're more likely to stay on your program. It only takes a moment—a small time investment, every day, to remind you of your commitment to a heart-healthy way of life.

STOCKING THE PANTRY WITH NUTRIENT-RICH FOODS

The TLC program emphasizes that, in making heart-healthy food choices, it's important to select low-calorie foods when possible—but that's not the only consideration. Although TLC doesn't explicitly require your to count all nutrients, it's always a good idea to pay attention to vitamins and minerals, and pass on those foods whose primary source of calories is sugar or fat. Women especially should take in 1,200 to 1,500 mg of calcium a day, either through healthy foods or by supplementation.

To get us in the right frame of mind for choosing overall-healthy foods, the National Cholesterol Education Program provides a list of healthier versions of some of our favorite foods. As we did in the previous chapter, we've modified the NCEP's list slightly to include more fresh, whole foods and eliminate processed foods and simple carbohydrates. The list includes:

Instead of:	Replace with:
Cheddar, Swiss, jack cheese	Reduced-calorie, low-fat cheese
American cheese	Fat-free American cheese
Ramen noodles	Brown rice or whole-grain noodles
Pasta with white/Alfredo sauce	Whole-grain pasta with red sauce (marinara)
Pasta with cheese sauce	Whole-grain pasta with vegetables (primavera)
Granola	Bran flakes
	Cooked oatmeal or grits
	Whole grains (such as couscous, barley, bulgur)
	Reduced-fat granola
Creamed soups	Low-sodium broth-based soups
Gravy (homemade with fat and/ or milk)	Au jus mixed with water
Avocado on sandwiches	Cucumber slices or lettuce leaves
Guacamole dip or refried beans with lard	Salsa
Cold cuts or lunch meats (such as bologna, salami, liverwurst)	Low-fat cold cuts (95–97% fat-free)

Hot dogs (regular)	Low-fat chicken or turkey sausage
Bacon or sausage	Canadian bacon or lean ham
Regular ground beef	Extra lean ground beef (such as ground round or ground turkey)
Beef (chuck, rib, brisket)	Beef (round, loin, trimmed of fat)
Croissants, brioches	Whole-grain rolls or breads
Donuts, sweet rolls, muffins, scones, pastries	Whole-grain English muffin with "just fruit" unsweetened fruit spread
Party crackers	Low-fat whole-grain, low-sodium crackers
Cake (pound, chocolate, yellow)	Cake (angel food)
Nuts	Air-popped or light microwave popcorn, fruits, vegetables
Ice cream	Sorbet, sherbet, fat-free frozen yogurt, frozen fruit
Custard or puddings made with whole milk	Sugar-free puddings made with skim milk

SHOPPING FOR THE BEST FATS

You learned in previous chapters that the amount of fat in an item isn't always as important as the *kind* of fats in that food. Some foods have high levels of trans fats, which everyone should try to avoid altogether—especially those who are aiming for healthy cholesterol—while other foods have no trans fats at all. We also need to pay attention to the amount of saturated, monounsaturated and polyunsaturated fat contents. Remember, it is the *saturated* fats, or foods that say "partially hydrogenated" oils or fats on the label, that along with trans fats will help raise your LDL levels.

Did you know that many kitchen shops now host olive oil tastings, just as wine stores offer wine tastings? If you haven't tasted the differences between oils, now is a good time to inform yourself, because you'll want to choose the "right" fats and oils for your heart-healthy diet—and much of the time, olive oil, which is 74 percent monounsaturated, will be your best choice.

These days, it's common practice for better restaurants to serve their homemade breads with seasoned olive oil instead of butter. Why not do this at home? You don't need to wait for company; simply pour a little high-quality olive oil into a small saucer, add some fresh-ground black pepper (and other herbs, if you like) and dip your artisanal whole-grain bread into the oil, bite by bite. It makes a wonderfully easy, tasty healthy appetizer.

You can also use olive oil in baking. A deli or market that specializes in oils can help you make good decisions about buying healthy oils. Many supermarkets and commercial brands—including Trader Joe's, Wegman's and Pam—even offer olive-oil-flavored cooking sprays, along with other flavors such as lemon and garlic. Also relatively healthy is canola oil, extracted from rapeseed (a member of the cabbage family), at 50 percent monounsaturated fats.

SMART SHOPPING FOR CARBS

It's not always easy to choose your grains wisely, because the food industry tries its best to confuse you, luring you to pick up "whole wheat" instead of "whole grains," and labeling some foods "high fiber" when they're not.

Here is the best wisdom out there for buying healthy grains and carbs:

- It isn't enough to look for the words "whole" or "whole grain," says the American Heart Association. Make sure the whole grain is listed first in the list of ingredients. If one of the first ingredients listed is "enriched flour," it isn't really whole-grain bread.

- When you buy cereal, look for cereal with at least 5 grams of fiber per serving. You've read in earlier chapters that fiber can cut your chances of developing inflammation and type 2 diabetes; the Physicians' Health Study found that doctors who ate high-fiber cereal (meaning 5 grams per serving) were 28 percent less likely to suffer heart failure over a twenty-four-year period.

• Oatmeal is generally more heart-healthy than most cold cereals, and old-fashioned oats are usually healthier than instant-cook packets. Oatmeal is higher in soluble fiber and helps lower cholesterol levels. The packets often contain added sugar and sodium—but not always. If you enjoy the convenience of cereal packets, read the labels and make the best choice for your lifestyle.

• Extra-fiber breads are healthier. The AHA recommends 25 grams of fiber a day to help lower cholesterol; some whole-grain English muffins provide as many as 8 grams of fiber per muffin, or about one-third of your daily requirement.

• Switch to whole-wheat pasta—but again, read the labels! Many pastas are labeled "whole wheat," but if the first ingredient listed is enriched flour, it isn't whole-grain at all. True whole wheat pasta doesn't lose its bran during the processing, so it will contain more fiber and other nutrients.

• Health food stores often carry pastas with even more healthy ingredients, such as oats and barley. These grains provide more soluble fiber than wheat, so presumably the pastas made from them will be healthier—but taste them before you buy a case.

• Brown rice is healthier than white rice, a "simple" carb that converts quickly to glucose in your body, boosts your blood sugar and is stored as fat. Brown rice is a complex carb with 4 grams of fiber per cup, compared to white rice's 1 gram.

- Don't overlook barley, the king of high-fiber grains. Add it to soup, stew, even oatmeal; its taste and texture adapt easily to many foods, and it is rich in soluble fiber, which helps to lower LDL cholesterol.

- Again, read the labels of all packaged foods you buy! One serving of Kellogg's Frosted Mini-Wheats, for instance, contains 6 grams of fiber, and the first ingredient listed is "whole grain wheat." That would seem to qualify it as a relatively healthy breakfast food, but the second ingredient listed is sugar, and the third is "high fructose corn syrup"—another form of sugar. So this cereal, while healthy for most people, might not be the wisest choice for people who must severely restrict their sugar intake. A better choice for them might be Kellogg's Oat Bran Flakes, with a bit less fiber per serving (4 grams) but only half the sugar (6 grams).

- Don't hesitate to scoop your grains from the bulk food bins at the supermarket or health food stores! You know the oats, beans, nuts, seeds and other bulk items won't have the sodium or sugar that you'd find in their canned or otherwise processed counterparts, and they're almost always more economical when you buy them in bulk. If you store them in airtight containers, they'll stay fresh for a very long time—even in humid climates, up to a year in the refrigerator.

BRINGING YOUR FAMILY ALONG ON YOUR TLC PLAN

You don't need to worry about cooking separate meals for you and your family when you follow TLC. A heart-healthy eating plan is good for everyone, whether they need to lower their cholesterol levels or they already enjoy good heart health.

You will want to talk with them, of course, because they will notice you're eating fewer fats or smaller portions than they're eating at mealtimes. You could make your TLC part of a weekly "family challenge" of meal planning: Ask them what they want for their next five or seven dinners, then challenge them to help you think of ways to make your portions healthier.

Any scrumptious, high-fat dinner can be made healthier, even pizza. You could make your portion a personal-size pizza made with whole-wheat flour, adorned with tomato sauce, low-fat cheese, low-fat chicken sausage and plenty of veggies.

A family "salad bar" can be fun, with everyone choosing their own seeds, nuts, fruits, cheeses and dressings. If your family enjoys Chinese food, try cooking a stir fry with the meat or chicken on the side, almost as a condiment. And if, on occasion, your family wants a high-fat, red meat dinner such as prime rib, simply serve yourself a smaller portion of the meat.

PARTIES, TLC-STYLE

Whether it's a baby shower, a tailgate party or a sedate dinner party, we might be tempted to eat unhealthy foods when we gather with friends over meals. But don't give up—there really are TLC strategies for getting through parties without starving or resigning yourself to eating "rabbit food"! Here are a few ideas for hosts and party-goers.

• If you're giving the party, set only one rule: no deep-fried foods. If you're attending someone else's party, follow the same rule: no deep-fried foods. It's a good rule to follow, in fact, for the rest of your life. If the only entrée at a party is fried chicken, allow yourself one piece with all the skin and fat removed, and fill up on side items.

• Set several matching dishes on the buffet table, and fill them with nutrient-packed nuts: almonds, walnuts, and unsalted sunflower or pumpkin seeds. For a delicious twist, fill a dish with peanuts—but invest in gourmet redskin peanuts, either unsalted or lightly salted. Make sure you leave the red skins on the nut meats; they're full of resveratrol, the same anti-aging substance that makes red wine healthy. With nuts as with wine, enjoy in moderation!

• Instead of a high-fat creamy dip, prepare hummus and serve it with whole grain bread and celery or carrot sticks. Hummus is also widely available as a prepared food in supermarkets. Hummus is basically chick peas, sesame tahini and a bit of lemon juice, often with heart-healthy olive oil added. If you make your own, add interest to the flavor by making one small batch with roasted red peppers stirred in, another with garlic and onions, and another with artichokes. Garnish with olives and flat parsley.

• This tip is stolen from Martha Stewart: For your next crudité platter, display the veggies vertically, in pretty glasses, instead of in the usual, predictable flat tray. Include stand-ups such as blanched asparagus, tall carrots and long bell pepper strips.

• Take your time at the buffet table. Make a "scouting" trip to the table before you fill your plate. Give yourself time to think about your choices.

• If you're going to a potluck dinner, make your contribution a low-fat item that you enjoy eating. That way, you know there will be at least one food you can eat.

• You've heard this one before, but eating before a party can save you from diet setbacks. It's not necessary to sit down to an entire meal beforehand, but eating a light sandwich, or munching a couple of "lite" string cheeses, will help you view the buffet table with indifference when you get to your party.

THE FIVE WORST SUPER BOWL PARTY FOODS

Just try naming a healthy Super Bowl party food—it doesn't exist! Apparently, high fat and high cholesterol content are requirements for any food items served that afternoon in January. Typically, we down chicken wings, pizzas and beer by the case, and leave the party two pounds heavier and a step closer to heart disease. In fact, recent research has found that even one high-fat meal can constrict the arteries, restrict the flow of blood for hours after the meal, and increase your risk of suffering a heart attack that same day.

Super Bowl Sunday is second only to Thanksgiving in the amount of food served, says the USDA.

Dietitians working with The Cancer Project have found that most popular foods bought from fast-food restaurants on Super Bowl Sunday are high in fat, saturated fat, calories, sodium and cholesterol. Some also include processed or grilled meats, which The Cancer Project says are linked to increased cancer risk. Their list of the five most unhealthy takeout or delivery foods we order on Super Bowl Sunday:

Food	Restaurant
Deep Dish MeatZZA Feast	Domino's Pizza
The Meats Pan Crust Pizza	Papa John's
Creamy Chicken Alfredo Baked Tuscani Pasta	Pizza Hut
Tuna Melt	Quiznos
Honey BBQ Wings	KFC

DINING OUT WITH TLC

When you decide to eat out, your first question always is, Where should we eat? You can narrow down your choices by avoiding chain restaurants when you can. A family-owned restaurant, or even a diner, often can be more flexible in preparing your meal the way you'd like. They can substitute ingredients, cooking a dish in broth instead of cream, for example, or grilling your favorite fish instead of frying it.

Then, most of us make the same mistake when we eat in restaurants: We don't ask about the food we're going to order—how it's prepared, what kinds of oils are used, whether it's made by the restaurant's chef or, more likely if it's a chain restaurant, at some massive food factory a thousand miles away and transported here by refrigerator truck.

You'll never know what's in a dish if you don't ask. There's no reason to give up your TLC plan when you go to a restaurant, and we've included a long list of tips to help you enjoy a meal that's both satisfying and healthy.

Before ordering

- Decide what you feel like eating before you leave your house. Challenge yourself to stick with that plan!

- Always ask for dressings, sauces and gravies on the side. A bit on your fork will give you all the creamy taste you need to enjoy your meal.

- Don't let anyone rush you through your decision. Take your time with the menu, just as you learned to do at a party buffet table.

- Ask the waiter to remove your butter and white bread. Don't be timid about asking if there is any whole-grain bread in the kitchen.

- Ask for a glass of water as soon as you're seated, and drink two or three full glasses throughout the meal.

- Don't order any foods that are fried, creamed or cooked in butter.

When you order

- Look for meals that are described as broiled, baked, steamed, roasted, stir fried or lightly sautéed.

- One of my favorite tricks: Order an appetizer instead of an entrée, and a side salad or cup of soup.

- If a dish comes with fries, ask if salad can be substituted.

- At Chinese restaurants, the healthier items will be steamed, roasted or poached—and if you do order a stir-fry, always ask that it be prepared with less oil than usual.

- At Italian restaurants, if you're ordering a pasta dish, choose red or broth sauces over creamy, or pasta simply tossed in olive oil and garlic.

- Avoid ordering lasagna, eggplant or chicken parmigiana. The cheese will likely add too many calories to the dish.

- At Mexican restaurants, choose rice and black beans, salsa and spicy chicken. Grilled chicken fajitas can be a good choice; skip the sour cream. And always, skip the deep-fried items.

- Most fast-food restaurants now offer salads, grilled chicken sandwiches with no breading, or roast beef sandwiches—but pay special attention to the ingredients and how the foods are prepared. In the restaurant nutrition counter that follows, you will find shockingly high calorie, fat and sodium counts for salads in some restaurants!

- Always keep an eye out for lower-fat items, such as minestrone soup instead of "creamy tomato" or roasted potatoes instead of fried.

- Never assume that a vegetable soup does not contain cream. Always ask.

- Skip dessert or if you must, order sorbet or fruit without toppings.

- When your food arrives, if the portion is a large one, divide the meal in half and take it home for lunch the next day.

- Remember to eat mindfully! If nothing else, put down your fork between bites; that step alone will slow you down and you will want to eat less.

IT'S ALL A MATTER OF BALANCE

This book has taken you through the science of cholesterol and a comprehensive look at how foods affect your cholesterol levels. You've learned a lot about reaching healthy HDL, LDL and triglyceride levels, and how you can design your own food plan to suit your healthy-cholesterol goals.

Of all the factors that contribute to a heart-healthy lifestyle, food is by far the most important—but it doesn't work alone. In the next chapter, you will read about nutritional supplements, and the ways in which many have been proven to support healthy cholesterol levels. Supplementation won't be everyone's choice, but for those who believe it might be helpful, we have included the most up-to-date information available on the impact that such substances as magnesium, calcium and vitamin C, along with many others, have on cholesterol levels.

Lastly, in Chapter 8 we will look at other important factors that can balance out our heart-healthy lifestyle, including exercise, meditation and other relaxation techniques, and importantly, not smoking.

First, however, we have included a nutrient counter, listing hundreds of the most popular foods ordered at chain restaurants. Many of these you'll never want to eat again, or you may order them on very rare occasions; we include them mostly as a reference to remind you of how easily we can slip back into unhealthy life choices. We also found it encouraging, as we were compiling this list, that we spotted so many healthy choices. There isn't a restaurant listed where you couldn't find a meal that supports your TLC goals.

So go out, enjoy your meal and *one* glass of wine, and use this counter as a quick reference before you decide where to eat.

RESTAURANT NUTRITION COUNTER

ARBY'S	Cals	Fat (g)	SatFat (g)
BREAKFAST			
Biscuit, plain	273	15	4
Ham/egg/cheese biscuit	444	26	8
Bacon/egg/cheese croissant	378	25	12
Ham/egg/cheese croissant	361	21	10
Sausage/egg croissant	433	32	13
Sausage/egg/chs croissant	475	35	15
French Toastix	312	13	2
Sausage patty	210	20	7
Breakfast syrup	78	0	0
SANDWICHES			
Beef 'n cheddar, med	536	27	9
Beef 'n cheddar, lg	657	36	12
Roast beef, lg	547	28	12
Roast beef, reg	320	14	5
Chicken/bacon/Swiss, crisp	544	25	7
Chicken cordon bleu, crisp	577	28	7
Chicken fillet, crispy	488	23	4
Chicken/bacon/Swiss, roast	439	18	6
Chicken fillet, roasted	383	16	3
Roast ham & Swiss	691	31	8
Roast turkey & Swiss	708	30	8

Sodium (mg)	Carbs (g)	Fiber (g)	Sugar (g)
786	28	1	3
1734	31	1	4
850	23	1	3
1138	1	4	19
784	23	1	3
982	23	1	3
491	44	1	11
480	0	0	0
25	20	0	11
1701	44	2	8
2309	46	3	8
1869	41	3	6
953	34	2	5
1632	50	2	9
1936	47	2	7
1210	47	2	6
1343	30	2	10
921	37	2	7
1952	75	5	19
1677	74	5	17

ARBY'S

	Cals	Fat (g)	SatFat (g)
SUBS			
French dip & Swiss toasted	533	19	8
Classic Italian toasted	596	27	7
Philly beef toasted	610	30	0
Turkey bacon club toasted	605	24	6
SIDES			
Cheddar fries, med	546	33	5
Curly fries, sm	338	20	4
Curly fries, med	496	29	5
Curly fries, lg	604	36	7
Mozzarella sticks, reg, 4	426	28	13
Potato cakes, 2	246	18	4
Arby's sauce	15	0	0
Horsey sauce	62	5	1
KIDS, DESSERTS			
Jr. roast beef sandwich	272	10	4
Curly fries	234	14	3
Apple turnover w/icing	380	14	7
Cherry turnover w/icing	364	13	7

AU BON PAIN

BREAKFAST			
Asiago cheese bagel	340	6	4
Cinnamon raisin bagel	320	1	0

Sodium (mg)	Carbs (g)	Fiber (g)	Sugar (g)
2169	67	3	3
1831	65	3	4
1549	62	3	3
1701	65	3	3
1525	62	6	0
791	39	4	0
1160	58	6	0
1413	70	7	0
1370	38	2	5
391	26	2	0
177	4	0	1
173	3	0	1
740	34	2	5
548	27	3	0
287	58	3	37
269	58	1	35
620	56	2	5
450	68	3	13

AU BON PAIN	Cals	Fats (g)	SatFat (g)
BREAKFAST			
Everything bagel	340	5	0
Honey 9 grain bagel	350	4	0
Plain bagel	280	1	0
Chocolate croissant	440	22	13
Ham/cheese croissant	400	20	11
Plain croissant	310	17	9
Blueberry muffin	490	17	2
Carrot walnut muffin	560	27	6
Corn muffin	490	17	3
Cranberry walnut muffin	540	25	3
Double choc chunk muffin	620	25	8
Low-fat triple berry muffin	620	25	8
Raisin bran muffin	480	11	2
Cinnamon scone	530	27	16
Orange scone	470	23	13
Egg on a bagel	360	4	1
Egg on a bagel w/bacon	420	8	3
Egg on bagel w/bacon/chs	510	15	6
Egg on a bagel w/cheese	450	10	5
Portobello, egg, cheddar	500	26	14
Sausage/egg/cheddar on Asiago bagel	810	47	23
French pecan toast, 1 oz	70	4	2
Roasted potatoes, 1 oz	50	5	2
Sausage w/pepper/ onions, 1 oz	50	5	2

Sodium (mg)	Carbs (g)	Fiber (g)	Sugar (g)
990	61	3	4
490	69	6	7
430	56	2	4
210	58	3	27
660	38	2	5
220	31	1	3
510	74	2	31
820	72	4	40
600	75	3	31
500	66	4	28
540	86	4	47
720	65	2	33
600	85	10	43
400	60	2	22
420	57	1	17
790	60	3	5
1000	60	3	5
1140	61	3	5
930	61	3	5
1160	42	3	2
1540	58	1	5
45	8	0	4
90	1	0	1
90	1	0	1

AU BON PAIN	Cals	Fats (g)	SatFat (g)
BREAKFAST			
Scrambled eggs, 1 oz	35	3	1
Oatmeal, sml	150	3	0
Blueberry yogurt w/blueberries, sml	250	3	2
Granola topping, 2 oz	230	8	1
Strawberry yogurt w/blueberries, sm	250	2	2
Vanilla yogurt w/blueberries, sm	220	3	2
SANDWICHES			
Tuna melt	690	30	10
Turkey club	700	31	13
Turkey melt	810	32	13
Ham & Swiss on country white bread	530	17	9
Roast beef & Brie on country style bread	600	21	11
Tuna & cheddar on country white bread	610	25	9
Turkey & Swiss on country white bread	530	14	8
SALADS			
Caesar Asiago salad	220	12	6
Chef's salad	250	15	7
Garden salad	70	2	0
Grilled chicken Caesar Asiago salad	300	13	6
Mandarin sesame chicken salad	310	17	1
Mediterranean chicken salad	290	16	6

Sodium (mg)	Carbs (g)	Fiber (g)	Sugar (g)
90	1	0	1
10	28	4	1
135	50	0	43
75	37	3	11
135	50	0	43
180	41	0	32
1160	71	5	5
1970	59	2	2
2040	79	3	16
1930	60	2	2
1290	59	3	2
1330	63	3	4
1410	60	2	2
480	18	3	4
1030	7	3	4
85	13	3	3
740	18	3	4
410	29	3	10
1230	12	3	2

AU BON PAIN	Cals	Fats (g)	SatFat (g)
SALADS			
Tuna garden salad	240	12	2
Turkey cobb salad	330	19	8
SOUP			
Beef & vegetable, sm	219	10	2
Black bean, sm	200	4	6
Broccoli cheddar, sm	200	14	6
Chicken Florentine, sm	170	8	4
Chicken noodle, sm	90	2	1
Clam chowder, sm	210	12	5
Corn chowder, sm	230	12	6
Cream of chicken & wild rice, sm	160	9	4
French Moroccan tomato lentil, sm	120	2	0
French onion, sm	80	3	1
Garden vegetable, sm	50	1	0
Gazpacho, sm	60	3	0
Italian wedding, sm	110	5	2
Old-fashioned tomato	130	5	2
Split pea w/ham, sm	170	1	0
Thai coconut curry, sm	110	5	1
Tomato basil bisque, sm	140	6	4
Tomato rice, sm	80	1	0
Vegetarian chili, sm	150	2	0
Wild mushroom bisque, sm	120	6	2
PASTA			
Meat lasagna, 10.7 oz	470	24	11
Macaroni & cheese, sm	330	19	2

Sodium (mg)	Carbs (g)	Fiber (g)	Sugar (g)
480	15	4	5
930	14	4	4
720	17	2	3
740	30	17	2
660	13	1	5
700	17	1	3
700	12	1	2
680	18	1	5
750	27	2	7
650	15	1	2
710	21	7	4
870	13	1	4
720	9	2	3
1020	8	2	4
870	13	2	3
770	18	2	10
810	28	10	2
700	14	1	4
330	18	2	10
190	16	1	4
650	26	13	3
680	15	2	4
1080	41	5	7
920	24	1	3

AU BON PAIN	Cals	Fats (g)	SatFat (g)
SIDES, SNACKS			
Apples, blue cheese & cranberries, 5 oz	200	10	4
Baked potato, 1 oz	25	0	0
Black bean & corn salad, 6 oz	130	0	0
Brie/fruit/crackers, 3.5 oz	200	11	6
Brown rice/hazelnut waldorf salad, 4.5 oz	180	9	2
Cheddar, fruit, crackers 3.5 oz	200	12	6
Chicken pesto salad	160	8	3
Choc. covered almonds	230	15	5
Creamed spinach, 1 oz	40	3	1
Fresh watermelon, 8 oz	70	0	0
Fruit cup, sm (6 oz)	200	7	2
Hummus & cucumber, 4.3 oz	130	8	0
Roasted apple cranberry orzo, 1 oz	45	1	0
DESSERTS			
Choc. cheesecake brownie	460	19	6
Chocolate chip cookie	280	13	7
Oatmeal raisin cookie	230	8	4
Pecan roll	810	41	14
Shortbread cookie	340	20	10
White chocolate chunk macadamia cookie	300	16	8

Sodium (mg)	Carbs (g)	Fiber (g)	Sugar (g)
270	27	3	21
20	5	1	0
310	25	5	2
280	18	0	9
160	22	2	8
280	18	0	9
420	1	1	1
10	20	2	17
90	1	0	1
0	17	1	4
15	18	1	15
460	10	3	1
25	9	1	3
400	74	1	50
210	40	2	24
190	36	2	23
430	99	3	47
300	37	1	11
240	36	1	21

AU BON PAIN	Cals	Fats (g)	SatFat (g)
BREAD			
Artisan baguette, sandwich size	310	3	1
Artisan baguette, salad size	230	2	1
Artisan honey multigrain baguette, sandwich size	340	5	0
Artisan honey multigrain baguette, salad size	250	3	0
Artisan sundried tomato bread, 4 oz	270	1	0
Asiago breadstick	190	4	3
Ciabatta, sm	180	1	0
Ciabatta, lg	310	1	0
Cinnamon raisin breadstick	190	1	0
Everything breadstick	170	3	0
Whole wheat multigrain bread	260	3	0
DRESSING/ CONDIMENTS			
Balsamic vinaigrette dressing, 2 oz	120	9	2
Blue cheese dressing, 2 oz	310	33	6
Caesar dressing, 2 oz	270	28	5
Fat-free raspberry vinaigrette, 2 oz	50	0	0
Hazelnut vinaigrette, 2 oz	270	25	4
Light ranch dressing, 2 oz	120	11	2

Sodium (mg)	Carbs (g)	Fiber (g)	Sugar (g)
760	61	2	1
570	46	2	1
670	66	6	1
500	49	4	1
750	57	2	2
350	28	1	3
480	38	2	1
820	64	3	2
230	41	2	13
500	31	1	2
630	53	9	4
360	8	0	8
460	2	0	2
370	4	0	2
190	12	0	12
300	11	0	10
410	3	0	2

AU BON PAIN

	Cals	Fats (g)	SatFat (g)
DRESSING/ CONDIMENTS			
Light honey mustard dressing, 2 oz	170	9	2
Light olive oil vinaigrette, 2 oz	110	10	2
Basil pesto, 1 oz	120	12	2
Chili Dijon, 1 oz	120	12	2
Guacamole, 1 oz	50	5	1
Herb mayonnaise, 1 oz	110	11	2'
Honey mustard sauce, 2.5 oz	200	3	0
Honey pecan cream cheese, 2 oz	200	16	0
Mustard, 1 tsp	0	0	0
Sun-dried tomato spread, 0.5 oz	45	4	0
BEVERAGE			
Caffe Americano, sm	5	0	0
Caffe latte, sm (12 oz)	200	11	7
Cappuccino, sm (12 oz)	120	7	4
Caramel macchiato, sm	350	10	6
Chai latte, sm (12 oz)	290	11	7
Mocha latte, sm (12 oz)	300	16	10

Auntie Anne's

	Cals	Fats (g)	SatFat (g)
PRETZELS			
Garlic pretzel	350	5	3
Garlic pretzel w/o butter	310	1	0
Original pretzel	340	5	3
Original pretzel w/o butter	310	1	0

Sodium (mg)	Carbs (g)	Fiber (g)	Sugar (g)
380	20	0	12
420	6	0	5
220	1	0	0
130	3	1	2
115	3	2	0
160	1	0	1
240	41	1	39
135	10	1	9
70	0	0	0
70	1	0	1
15	1	0	1
170	17	0	17
85	10	0	10
160	53	0	50
130	38	0	26
160	35	1	33
990	65	2	10
990	65	2	10
1060	63	2	9
990	65	2	10

Auntie Anne's	Cals	Fats (g)	SatFat (g)
PRETZELS			
Pretzel pocket, bacon/ egg/cheese	580	23	10
Pretzel pocket, pepperoni	650	27	12
Pretzel pocket, turkey/ cheddar	470	10	5
Sesame pretzel	400	10	3.5
Sesame pretzel w/o butter	360	6	1
Sour cream/onion pretzel	360	5	3
Sour cream/onion pretzel w/o butter	330	1.5	0
Cinnamon sugar pretzel	470	12	7
Cinnamon sugar pretzel w/o butter	380	1	0

Bob Evans			
EGGS			
Border scramble omelet	621	44	18
Border scramble omelet, B.Evans egg lites	441	25	13
Farmer's Market omelet	621	43	21
Farmer's Market omelet, B.Evans egg lites	440	25	16
Garden Harvest omelet	503	34	17
Garden Harvest omelet, B.Evans egg lites	323	16	12
Ham & cheddar omelet	477	33	13
Ham & cheddar omelet, B.Evans egg lites	296	14	8

Sodium (mg)	Carbs (g)	Fiber (g)	Sugar (g)
790	71	2	12
1120	75	2	11
1050	73	2	14
990	67	3	10
990	67	3	10
1180	68	2	12
1180	68	2	12
400	84	2	29
400	84	2	29
1569	16	3	9
1248	15	3	9
2209	14	1	6
1888	13	1	6
1726	14	2	6
1405	13	2	6
1773	4	0	2
1451	3	0	2

Bob Evans	Cals	Fats (g)	SatFat (g)
EGGS			
Sausage & cheddar omelet	640	49	19
Sausage & cheddar omelet, B.Evans egg lites	459	31	14
Spinach, bacon & tomato country benedict	760	51	17
Three cheese omelet	490	37	17
Three cheese omelet, B.Evans egg lites	309	18	12
Turkey & spinach omelet	580	37	16
Turkey & spinach omelet, B.Evans egg lites	400	18	11
Western omelet	487	32	13
Western omelet, B.Evans egg lites	310	14	8
HOTCAKES			
Blueberry w/o topping, 1	343	10	2
Buttermilk w/o topping, 1	337	10	2
Cinnamon w/o topping, 1	382	12	4
Multigrain w/o topping, 1	374	11	4
Stacked & stuffed blueberry cream hotcakes	1047	36	16
Stacked & stuffed cinnamon cream hotcakes	1070	43	20

Sodium (mg)	Carbs (g)	Fiber (g)	Sugar (g)
1538	4	0	2
1217	3	0	2
1972	43	1	8
1415	4	0	2
1094	3	0	2
2386	7	1	5
2065	6	1	5
1744	7	1	4
1453	6	1	4
792	58	2	18
792	56	2	16
792	62	2	22
897	61	4	18
1852	165	6	80
1911	155	4	72

Bob Evans	Cals	Fats (g)	SatFat (g)
SPECIALTY BREAKFAST			
Country biscuit breakfast	666	46	16
Fit from the Farm breakfast w/parfait	306	4	1
Fit from the Farm breakfast w/oatmeal	347	6	2
Fit from the Farm breakfast w/yogurt crepe	495	15	5
Turkey sausage breakfast	362	7	2
BREAKFAST SIDE/ CONDIMENT			
Apple butter, 0.5 oz	34	0	2
Bacon, 1 pc	36	4	2
Banana nut bread	215	8	1
Beef gravy, 2.2 oz	25	1	0
Biscuit	274	14	4
Blueberry bread	261	12	2
Bowl of oatmeal	167	3	0
Cinnamon swirl, frosted	532	28	0
Country gravy, 3 oz	56	4	1
Cup of grits	148	6	2
Pancake syrup, 3 oz	213	0	0
Sausage patty, 1	140	11	4
Sausage link, 1	133	12	3
Smoked ham, 1 pc	99	3	1
Sugar-free pancake syrup, 3 oz	39	0	0
Turkey sausage, 1 pc	72	4	1

Sodium (mg)	Carbs (g)	Fiber (g)	Sugar (g)
1697	39	0	6
703	41	3	36
813	46	3	29
933	61	6	41
1009	48	5	18
2	8	0	7
54	0	0	0
125	34	2	21
419	3	0	0
885	32	0	3
338	36	1	20
259	31	4	1
602	67	0	21
303	6	0	2
143	22	1	0
101	55	0	44
313	0	0	0
184	0	0	0
1293	3	0	1
79	10	0	0
404	1	0	0

Bob Evans	Cals	Fats (g)	SatFat (g)
SALAD			
Chili & cheese taco salad	855	64	18
Cobb salad	568	37	18
Country Caesar salad	746	53	12
Country spinach salad	479	31	8
Cranberry pecan chicken salad	894	60	17
Garden salad	58	1	0
Specialty garden salad	124	7	3
Wildfire fried chicken salad	711	34	9
Wildfire grilled chicken salad	440	19	6
SOUP, CHILI			
Bean soup, cup	110	2	1
Bean soup, bowl	204	4	1
Cheddar baked potato soup, cup	172	9	6
Cheddar baked potato soup, bowl	242	13	8
Veg. beef soup, cup	90	2	1
Veg. beef soup, bowl	135	3	1
Sausage chili, cup	215	14	4
Sausage chili, bowl	351	22	8
SANDWICH			
Bob's BLT&E	639	41	15
Bob's-B-Q pulled pork	599	25	4
Chicken salad, half	319	19	3

Sodium (mg)	Carbs (g)	Fiber (g)	Sugar (g)
1565	52	11	10
1673	10	3	4
1712	20	1	4
1297	12	5	4
2338	45	5	34
132	9	1	2
334	10	1	2
1332	70	7	18
963	37	6	14
549	15	4	0
1016	28	8	1
744	15	0	2
1046	22	1	3
503	13	2	6
759	20	3	8
550	15	6	1
898	24	9	2
1021	26	3	7
741	67	4	26
646	27	3	6

Bob Evans	Cals	Fats (g)	SatFat (g)
SANDWICH			
Fried chicken club	637	31	11
Fried chicken sandw.	489	18	4
Fried haddock	732	33	10
Grilled cheese	350	15	6
Grilled chicken club	583	31	11
Grilled chicken sandw.	441	19	4
Pot roast sandw., half	371	18	7
Turkey bacon melt, half	292	14	6
BURGER			
Bacon cheeseburger	719	38	17
Cheeseburger	648	31	13
Hamburger	542	22	8
ENTRÉE			
Country fried steak	496	33	11
Ital. sausage/pepper pasta	696	40	12
Meatloaf	435	22	8
Open-faced roast beef	476	24	8
Sirloin steak	421	29	9
Steak tips & noodles	266	15	4
Bob-B-Q roasted chicken	326	14	4
Chicken parmesan	691	28	9
Chicken salad plate	712	43	6
Fried chicken breast	285	12	3
Fried chicken strips, 1 pc	137	8	1
Garlic butter grilled chicken breast	242	14	3

Sodium (mg)	Carbs (g)	Fiber (g)	Sugar (g)
1567	47	3	4
1109	47	3	4
1596	71	4	6
729	22	2	4
1420	34	2	4
971	33	2	4
829	30	2	8
1035	23	1	3
1355	35	2	5
1247	35	2	5
776	34	2	4
1217	31	0	0
2001	54	5	13
1958	22	1	11
1041	22	1	9
638	3	0	0
828	3	0	0
1151	15	1	15
2365	65	5	13
974	70	12	56
758	13	1	0
301	10	0	0
691	1	0	0

Bob Evans	Cals	Fats (g)	SatFat (g)
ENTRÉE			
Pork Bob-B-Q ribs	377	13	5
Pork Bob-B-Q ribs dinner	759	26	10
Fried haddock	363	18	4
Garden vegetable alfredo	809	48	20
Garden vegetable & salmon alfredo	975	54	20
Garlic butter salmon	300	15	3
Potato-crusted flounder	218	12	3
Salmon stir-fry	760	28	5
Salmon	294	14	3
Vegetable stir-fry	507	14	2
SIDES			
Applesauce	69	0	0
Baked potato	220	3	0
Broccoli florets	44	1	0
Coleslaw	208	14	2
Corn	166	11	4
Corn & pepper relish	16	0	0
Cottage cheese	92	4	2
Cranberry relish	68	0	0
Dinner roll	201	5	1
French fries	319	13	3
Glazed carrots	75	3	1
Green beans	47	2	1
Home fries	183	6	1
Loaded baked potato	388	16	8
Mashed potatoes	192	7	4
Onion petals	301	18	2
Rice pilaf	133	5	1

Sodium (mg)	Carbs (g)	Fiber (g)	Sugar (g)
937	38	2	27
1889	77	5	54
608	27	2	2
1860	72	10	14
1715	60	6	10
172	1	0	0
531	9	0	1
2126	78	6	27
101	0	0	0
2050	87	9	31
11	18	2	13
525	51	6	6
41	8	5	3
243	19	1	17
258	17	2	2
2	4	1	1
310	4	1	3
7	16	1	15
268	34	1	6
92	46	1	0
85	13	3	6
515	6	2	1
685	28	3	14
983	53	6	7
428	16	1	1
464	35	2	3
620	21	1	1

Bob Evans	Cals	Fats (g)	SatFat (g)
DESSERTS & TOPPINGS			
Coconut cream pie	528	28	19
French silk pie	662	44	26
Oreo ice cream pie	883	42	19
Strawberry shortcake	569	22	11
Strawberry Supreme pie	651	47	22
Blueberry topping, 3 oz	103	0	0
Caramel topping, 1 oz	74	0	0
Chocolate fudge topping, 1 oz	86	2	1

Boston Market			
INDIVIDUAL MEALS			
Meatloaf	520	36	16
Chicken, 3 pc dark	390	22	6
Chicken, ¼ white rotisserie	320	12	4
Chicken, ¼ white rotisserie w/o skin	240	4	1
Half rotisserie chicken	610	29	9
1 thigh & 1 drumstick	290	17	5
Pastry top chicken pot pie	800	48	18
Roasted turkey	150	2.5	1
SOUP/SIDES			
Baked beans	270	1.5	0
Caesar side salad w/o dressing	40	2	1.5

Sodium (mg)	Carbs (g)	Fiber (g)	Sugar (g)
423	64	4	41
320	60	2	44
692	121	3	44
924	86	4	49
333	58	3	40
14	25	2	23
79	18	0	14
46	16	0	11
1030	21	0	4
1270	1	0	1
900	0	0	0
890	1	0	0
1860	1	0	1
950	0	0	1
1090	59	4	4
500	0	0	0
1000	53	11	13
75	3	1	1

Boston Market	Cals	Fat (g)	SatFat (g)
SOUP/SIDES			
Chicken noodle soup	250	8	2.5
Cinnamon apples	210	3	0
Coleslaw	300	20	4.5
Creamed spinach	280	23	15
Fresh steamed vegetables	60	2	0
Garlic dill new potatoes	140	3	1
Green beans	60	3.5	1.5
Macaroni & cheese	300	11	7
Mashed potatoes	270	11	5
Poultry gravy, 4 oz	50	2	0.5
Beef gravy, 3 oz	35	1.5	0.5
Potato salad	390	29	7
Seasonal fresh fruit salad	60	0	0
Sweet corn	170	4	1
Sweet potato casserole	460	16	4.5
SANDWICHES			
Rotisserie chicken open-faced	320	8	2.5
Roasted turkey open-faced	330	6	1.5
Meatloaf open-faced	670	38	17
Classic chicken salad	800	41	7
Boston Chicken Carver, half	375	14.5	4
Boston Turkey Carver, half	350	13	4
Boston Meatloaf Carver	980	46	21
Crispy Country Chicken Carver	1020	42	7

Sodium (mg)	Carbs (g)	Fiber (g)	Sugar (g)
1420	23	2	2
15	47	3	42
280	27	4	22
580	12	4	1
40	8	3	3
120	24	3	2
180	7	3	1
1100	35	2	6
820	36	4	2
690	7	0	2
500	4	0	0
640	26	3	1
20	15	1	13
95	37	2	10
270	77	3	39
1630	34	1	6
1480	43	1	14
1760	48	1	7
1900	65	4	5
980	32	1	2
850	32	2	2
2350	92	4	12
2210	114	4	23

Boston Market	Cals	Fat (g)	SatFat (g)
DESSERTS			
Chocolate chip fudge brownie	320	13	3
Cornbread	180	5	1.5

Bruegger's

	Cals	Fat (g)	SatFat (g)
BREAKFAST			
Asiago parmesan bagel	330	20	3
Blueberry bagel	320	2	0
Chocolate chip bagel	350	5	1.5
Cinnamon raisin bagel	330	2	0
Everything bagel	310	2	0
Fortified multigrain bagel	350	4	0
Garlic bagel	320	2	0
Honey grain bagel	330	3	0
Onion bagel	320	2	0
Plain bagel	300	2	0
Poppy bagel	310	2.5	0
Pumpernickel bagel	330	2.5	0
Rosemary olive oil bagel	350	7	0
Sesame bagel	310	3	0
Sourdough bagel	310	2	0
Sundried tomato bagel	320	2	0
Whole wheat bagel	390	6	0
Asiago parmesan square bagel	360	4.5	1.5
Everything square bagel	320	2	0
Breakfast bagel w/ bacon & plain bagel	460	23	8

Sodium (mg)	Carbs (g)	Fiber (g)	Sugar (g)
220	49	3	36
320	31	0	12
670	61	4	7
530	67	3	14
570	64	4	14
510	69	4	17
790	31	4	7
550	69	6	10
560	65	4	8
510	65	5	10
560	64	4	8
620	60	4	7
620	61	4	7
620	67	5	11
540	64	4	10
620	61	4	7
570	63	4	7
640	64	4	11
680	73	9	8
740	66	4	11
740	64	4	8
980	65	4	9

Bruegger's	Cals	Fats (g)	SatFat (g)
BREAKFAST			
Breakfast bagel w/ ham & plain bagel	460	18	6
Breakfast bagel w/ sausage & plain bagel	640	30	11
Spinach/cheddar/ bacon omelet, sesame bagel	550	22	8
Spinach/cheddar/ham omelet, sesame bagel	540	17	7
Spinach/cheddar/ sausage omelet, sesame bagel	660	32	12
SANDWICHES			
BLT on plain bagel	570	23	5
Chicken breast on plain bagel	660	11	2.5
Garden veggie on plain bagel	400	2.5	0
Ham on plain bagel	410	5	1
Roast beef on plain bagel	730	39	5
Tuna salad on plain bagel	620	27	3.5
Turkey on plain bagel	510	14	1.5
Ham/Swiss panini on honey wheat	600	18	8
Tuna/cheddar melt panini on honey wheat	1020	67	15
Herby turkey sandwich on sesame bagel	600	14	4.5
Leonardo de Veggie on Asiago Softwich	590	17	9

Sodium (mg)	Carbs (g)	Fiber (g)	Sugar (g)
1270	73	4	11
1360	63	4	8
1290	60	3	8
1140	65	4	10
970	64	4	8
1060	72	5	10
780	87	5	26
620	82	7	14
1780	66	4	12
1280	71	5	10
990	73	5	10
1290	70	5	9
1650	71	2	22
1560	61	3	9
1420	80	5	14
1120	83	7	19

Bruegger's	Cals	Fats (g)	SatFat (g)
SANDWICHES			
Tarragon chicken salad on hearty white	770	41	6
Turkey chipotle club on honey wheat	800	51	7
Roma roast beef on hearty white	770	44	12
SOUP & CHILI			
Butternut squash soup	240	17	9
Chicken wild rice soup	280	22	10
Fire roasted tomato soup	130	6	3
Four cheese broccoli soup	260	20	10
New England clam chowder	230	14	4.5
Spinach & lentil soup	110	3.5	1
Beef chili	190	8	3
White chicken chili	240	9	0

Chick-fil-A			
BREAKFAST			
Bacon/egg/cheese biscuit	490	26	12
Plain biscuit	310	13	6
Biscuit & gravy	420	20	8
Chicken biscuit	450	20	8
Chicken/egg/cheese bagel	500	20	6
Cinnamon cluster	400	15	6

Sodium (mg)	Carbs (g)	Fiber (g)	Sugar (g)
1370	73	3	5
1840	57	3	8
1740	62	3	6
650	21	1	2
840	12	1	2
920	17	2	10
1240	12	1	2
600	16	trace	12
570	16	7	2
880	18	6	3
630	26	7	2
1350	43	2	6
700	41	2	4
1370	51	2	5
1310	48	3	5
1280	49	3	9
280	61	3	28

Chick-fil-A	Cals	Fat (g)	SatFat (g)
BREAKFAST			
Hash browns	280	19	4
Sausage biscuit	590	41	16
Sausage breakfast burrito	480	27	11
SANDWICHES/ NUGGETS			
Chargrilled chicken club	380	12	5
Chargrilled chicken sandwich	260	3	0.5
Chicken salad sandwich	500	20	3.5
Chicken-n-Strips, 1 pc	120	6	1
Nuggets, 12	400	19	4
SALADS			
Chargrilled & fruit salad	220	6	3.5
Chargrilled chicken garden	170	6	3.5
Chick-n-Strips salad	450	22	6
SIDES			
Side salad	70	4.5	3
Carrot & raisin salad, sm	260	12	1.5
Cole slaw, sm	360	31	5
Fruit cup, sm	50	0	0
Waffle potato fries, sm	280	16	3.5
Waffle potato fries, med	370	21	4.5
Waffle potato fries, lg	420	24	5

Sodium (mg)	Carbs (g)	Fiber (g)	Sugar (g)
410	25	2	0
1250	42	4	2
870	38	4	3
1650	34	7	10
1300	33	7	9
1220	53	4	13
350	6	1	1
1250	15	3	4
860	21	4	16
860	10	4	5
1160	26	6	7
110	5	2	2
160	39	4	31
280	19	3	16
0	13	1	11
80	31	4	0
105	41	5	0
120	46	6	0

Chick-fil-A	Cals	Fat (g)	SatFat (g)
DESSERTS			
Cheesecake	310	23	13
Chocolate milkshake, sml	600	23	14
Cookies & cream milkshake, sm	570	26	14
Fudge nut brownie	370	19	6
Icedream, cup	290	7	4.5
Icedream, cone	170	4	2
Lemon pie	360	13	6
Peach milkshake, sm	720	19	11
Strawberry milkshake, sm	610	23	13
Vanilla milkshake, sm	540	23	13

Chili's			
APPETIZERS, WINGS			
Bottomless tostada chips w/hot sauce	470	39	5
Hos spinach/artichoke dip w/chips	930	77	34
Texas cheese fries w/Jalapeño ranch, full	1920	147	63
Triple Dipper chicken Crisper bites, 2	690	40	9
Triple Dipper buffalo chkn Crisper bites, 2	620	34	8
Triple Dipper boneless sweet chile glazed wings w/ranch, 5	760	50	9
Triple Dipper boneless buffalo wings w/bleu cheese, 5	740	60	10

Sodium (mg)	Carbs (g)	Fiber (g)	Sugar (g)
280	22	1	14
410	88	1	85
430	80	0	75
180	45	3	28
200	50	0	49
115	31	0	25
290	58	1	21
450	125	1	118
410	92	1	83
400	74	0	73
2790	28	5	na
3130	39	3	na
3570	67	7	na
1970	58	2	na
2380	54	2	na
1640	49	1	na
2070	26	1	na

Chili's	Cals	Fat (g)	SatFat (g)
APPETIZERS, WINGS			
Boneless buffalo wings w/bleu cheese	1200	91	15
SALADS			
Quesadilla explosion salad w/dressing	1270	76	23
Spicy garlic & lime grilled shrimp salad w/dressing	630	40	11
Mesquite chicken salad w/dressing	960	62	18
Chicken Caesar salad w/dressing	900	71	13
Southwestern Cobb salad w/dressing	1080	71	16
Side house salad w/o dressing	210	12	6
Side Caesar dressing w/dressing	350	31	6
SOUPS			
Broccoli cheese, cup	120	8	3.5
Chicken enchilada, cup	220	13	5
Chicken noodle, cup	60	0.5	0
New England clam chowder, cup	190	13	7
Southwestern veg., cup	100	4	1.5
SANDWICHES			
Bacon burger	1090	69	21
Big Mouth bites	1580	97	28
Mushroom-Swiss burger	1070	67	18

Sodium (mg)	Carbs (g)	Fiber (g)	Sugar (g)
3750	48	1	na
2650	86	10	na
1850	43	9	na
2680	45	10	na
1740	28	6	na
2650	57	9	na
310	17	3	na
550	13	2	na
650	9	1	na
690	9	1	na
580	10	1	na
390	11	1	na
630	13	2	na
1800	57	3	na
2930	104	6	na
1670	65	4	na

Chili's

	Cals	Fat (g)	SatFat (g)
SANDWICHES			
Jalapeño Smokehouse bacon Bigmouth burger	1690	120	39
Southern Smokehouse bacon Bigmouth burger	1630	108	36
Smokehouse bacon triple cheese Bigmouth burger	1750	123	44
Guiltless black bean burger	610	11	2
Cajun chicken sandwich	930	49	12
Chili's cheesesteak	880	44	17
Smoked turkey	960	55	14
Guiltless buffalo chicken	390	7	2
Guiltless grilled chicken	360	5	2
Fajita pita chicken	460	13	2
Chicken Caesar pita	700	41	8
ENTRÉES			
Spicy garlic/lime grilled chicken	170	11	2
Guiltless cedar plank tilapia	200	4	1
Guiltless honey-mustard glazed salmon	420	20	6
Guiltless grilled salmon	400	20	6
Guiltless chicken platter	370	2	1

Sodium (mg)	Carbs (g)	Fiber (g)	Sugar (g)
4050	68	4	na
4170	80	4	na
3860	66	3	na
1790	91	18	na
2400	70	40	na
1820	61	3	na
1790	57	2	na
2300	46	9	na
1390	44	9	na
1400	52	3	na
1570	45	4	na
1090	7	0	na
690	8	5	na
610	13	2	na
420	8	3	na
1940	49	7	na

Chili's

	Cals	Fat (g)	SatFat (g)
ENTRÉES			
Original ribs	990	68	25
Honey-chipotle ribs	1270	67	25
Honey BBQ ribs	1120	68	25
Cajun chicken pasta	1340	68	37
Monterey chicken	860	43	15
Margarita grilled chicken	680	14	2
Chicken tacos, 3	1200	45	17
Grilled shrimp alfredo	1320	76	38
Grilled salmon/garlic/ herbs	630	28	7
Country-fried steak w/toast & sides	1430	82	15
Classic chicken quesadilla	370	11	15
Fajita trio	560	27	5
Fire grilled chicken fajita quesadilla	1480	96	35
SIDES			
Rice & Kettle black beans	300	1.5	0
Spicy garlic/lime shrimp, 3	70	4.5	1
Cinnamon apples w/butter	190	7	2.5
Corn on the cob	190	7	1
Homestyle fries	410	25	4.5
Loaded mashed potatoes	390	25	8
Seasonal Veggies	60	4	1

Sodium (mg)	Carbs (g)	Fiber (g)	Sugar (g)
4100	33	2	na
4560	110	0	na
4780	66	2	na
3650	106	6	na
3060	57	9	na
2430	82	9	na
4430	144	16	na
3560	105	6	na
1050	50	5	na
2950	122	9	na
2000	25	4	na
3060	29	4	na
3510	99	6	na
1270	62	7	na
400	2	0	na
65	34	4	na
120	32	3	na
240	41	4	na
910	29	5	na
170	7	3	na

Chili's	Cals	Fat (g)	SatFat (g)
DESSERTS			
Cheesecake	700	42	26
Molten chocolate cake	1010	51	27
Sweet Shot key lime pie	240	12	8
Sweet Shot red velvet cake	250	9	4.5

Cinnabon

Classic Cinnabon	813	32	8
Cinnabon Stix	410	23	6
Cinnabon pretzel	750	6	2
Cinnabon Bites, 6	520	16	4
Pecanbon Bites, 4	670	28	7

Donatos

THIN CRUST PIZZA, ¼ OF LARGE			
Pepperoni	627	34	15
Serious Cheese	627	34	16
The Works	689	37	15
Vegy	544	24	11
Serious Meat	736	42	17
Spinach	611	34	16
Chicken spinach mozzarella	643	34	14
THICKER CRUST PIZZA, ¼ OF LARGE			
Pepperoni	798	39	16
Serious Cheese	798	38	17

Sodium (mg)	Carbs (g)	Fiber (g)	Sugar (g)
460	67	0	na
760	131	5	na
75	30	0	na
200	39	1	na
801	117	4	55
420	46	1	16
860	156	8	46
530	78	2	25
640	97	3	51
1471	50	2	9
1543	51	2	9
1716	56	4	11
1675	57	4	13
1973	52	3	10
1306	51	2	9
1367	49	2	10
1740	76	4	4
1812	77	4	4

Donatos

	Cals	Fat (g)	SatFat (g)
THICKER CRUST PIZZA, ¼ OF LARGE			
The Works	847	41	16
Vegy	715	29	12
Serious Meat	907	47	18
Chicken spinach mozzarella	803	39	15
HAND TOSSED PIZZA, 2 SLICES			
Pepperoni	499	27	12
Serious Cheese	597	25	14
The Works	669	31	14
Vegy	550	19	10
Serious Meat	735	37	16
Chicken spinach mozzarella	701	34	15
FLATBREAD PIZZA, WHOLE			
3 Meat	689	31	13
Cheese	693	31	15
Deluxe	613	25	10
Pepperoni	716	34	14
Vegy	606	24	10

Dunkin' Donuts

	Cals	Fat (g)	SatFat (g)
DONUTS			
Apple crumb	460	14	8
Apple 'n spice	240	11	4.5
Bavarian Kreme	250	12	5
Boston Kreme	280	12	5
Chocolate coconut cake	400	22	11

Sodium (mg)	Carbs (g)	Fiber (g)	Sugar (g)
1948	81	6	6
1944	83	6	7
2241	78	4	5
1482	73	3	4
1439	85	5	20
1324	65	5	10
1622	68	6	11
1489	70	6	12
1907	66	5	10
1061	61	4	8
1873	67	5	7
1773	66	5	7
1588	68	5	8
1775	67	5	7
1877	69	5	7
330	80	2	49
320	32	1	8
330	31	1	9
350	38	1	16
410	49	2	30

Dunkin' Donuts	Cals	Fat (g)	SatFat (g)
DONUTS			
Chocolate frosted cake	340	19	8
Chocolate glazed cake	280	15	7
Chocolate Kreme filled	310	16	7
Glazed	220	9	4
Jelly filled	260	11	5
French cruller	250	20	9
Apple fritter	400	15	6
Éclair	350	14	5
Glazed fritter	400	15	6
Plain cake stick	300	20	9
Glazed cake stick	400	20	9
DANISH/MUFFIN/ BISCUIT			
Apple cheese Danish	330	16	7
Cheese Danish	330	17	8
Blueberry muffin	510	16	1.5
Reduced fat blueberry muffin	450	10	1.5
Chocolate chip muffin	630	23	6
Corn muffin	510	17	2
English muffin	160	1.5	0
BREAKFAST ENTRÉE			
Egg & cheese on English muffin	320	13	5
Egg & cheese on bagel	480	15	5
Egg & cheese on croissant	470	28	12

Sodium (mg)	Carbs (g)	Fiber (g)	Sugar (g)
330	38	1	19
400	33	1	16
340	37	1	17
320	31	1	12
330	36	1	6
105	18	0	10
530	63	2	22
460	53	1	22
530	63	2	22
300	38	1	20
320	54	1	20
270	41	1	18
270	39	1	17
490	87	3	51
670	86	3	45
520	98	5	59
860	84	2	36
340	31	2	2
730	34	2	3
1180	75	3	2
750	39	1	6

Dunkin' Donuts	Cals	Fat (g)	SatFat (g)
BREAKFAST ENTRÉE			
Egg & cheese on biscuit	430	26	13
Ham/egg/cheese on English muffin	350	15	6
Ham/egg/cheese on bagel	520	17	6
Ham/egg/cheese on croissant	510	30	12
Ham/egg/cheese on biscuit	470	28	14
Bacon/egg/cheese on English muffin	360	16	6
Bacon/egg/cheese on bagel	530	18	6
Bacon/egg/cheese on croissant	510	31	13
Bacon/egg/cheese on biscuit	470	29	14
Sausage/egg/cheese on English muffin	490	28	10
Sausage/egg/cheese on bagel	660	29	11
Sausage/egg/cheese on croissant	640	42	17
Sausage/egg/cheese on biscuit	600	40	18
Supreme omelet & cheese on English muffin	350	15	7
Supreme omelet & cheese on bagel	520	17	7

Sodium (mg)	Carbs (g)	Fiber (g)	Sugar (g)
1010	36	1	4
1040	35	2	3
1480	75	3	2
1050	39	1	6
1320	36	1	4
920	35	2	4
1370	76	3	2
930	39	1	6
1200	36	1	4
1130	35	2	3
1590	76	3	2
1150	40	1	6
1410	37	1	4
1040	36	3	3
1480	77	3	2

Dunkin' Donuts

	Cals	Fat (g)	SatFat (g)
BREAKFAST ENTRÉE			
Supreme omelet & cheese on croissant	500	30	14
Supreme omelet & cheese on biscuit	470	28	15

McDonald's

	Cals	Fat (g)	SatFat (g)
BREAKFAST			
Egg McMuffin	300	12	5
Sausage McMuffin	370	22	8
Sausage McMuffin w/egg	450	27	10
English Muffin	160	3	0.5
Sausage biscuit w/egg	510	33	14
Sausage biscuit	430	27	12
Bacon/egg/cheese biscuit	420	23	12
Bacon/egg/cheese McGriddles	420	18	8
Sausage/egg/cheese McGriddles	560	32	12
Big breakfast, reg	740	48	17
Deluxe breakfast, reg	1090	56	19
Sausage burrito	300	16	7
Sausage patty	170	15	5
Scrambled eggs, 2	170	11	4
Hash brown	150	9	1.5
Hotcakes	350	9	2
Hotcakes & sausage	520	24	7
Hotcake syrup, 60 g	180	0	0

Sodium (mg)	Carbs (g)	Fiber (g)	Sugar (g)
1050	41	2	6
1310	37	2	4
820	30	2	3
850	29	2	2
920	30	2	2
280	27	2	2
1170	36	2	2
1080	34	2	2
1160	37	2	3
1110	48	2	15
1360	48	2	15
1560	51	3	3
2150	111	6	17
830	26	1	2
340	1	0	0
180	1	0	0
310	15	2	0
590	60	3	14
930	61	3	14
20	45	0	32

McDonald's	Cals	Fat (g)	SatFat (g)
SANDWICHES			
Hamburger	250	9	3.5
Cheeseburger	300	12	6
Double cheeseburger	440	23	11
Quarter Pounder	410	19	7
Quarter Pounder w/cheese	510	26	12
Big Mac	540	29	10
Filet-O-Fish	380	18	3.5
CHICKEN			
Chicken McNuggets, 4 pc	190	12	2
Chicken McNuggets, 6 pc	280	17	3
Chicken McNuggets, 10 pc	460	29	5
Chicken Selects Premium Breast Strips, 3	400	24	3.5
FRENCH FRIES			
French fries, sm	230	11	1.5
French fries, med	380	19	2.5
French fries, lg	500	25	3.5
SALADS			
Southwest salad w/grilled chicken	320	9	3
Southwest salad w/crispy chicken	430	20	4
Bacon ranch salad w/grilled chicken	260	9	4
Bacon ranch salad w/crispy chicken	370	20	6

Sodium (mg)	Carbs (g)	Fiber (g)	Sugar (g)
520	31	2	6
750	33	2	6
1150	34	2	7
730	37	2	8
1190	40	3	9
1040	45	3	9
640	28	2	5
400	11	0	0
600	16	0	0
1000	27	0	
1010	23	0	0
160	29	3	0
270	48	5	0
350	63	6	0
960	30	6	11
920	38	6	12
1010	12	3	5
970	20	3	6

McDonald's

	Cals	Fat (g)	SatFat (g)
SALADS			
Caesar salad w/grilled chicken	220	6	3
Snack size fruit & walnut salad	210	8	1.5
DESSERT			
Chocolate triple thick shake, 12 oz	440	10	6
Strawberry triple thick shake, 12 oz	420	10	6
Vanilla triple thick shake, 12 oz	420	10	6
Baked hot apple pie	250	13	7
Cinnamon melts	460	19	9

Panera Bread

	Cals	Fat (g)	SatFat (g)
BREAKFAST			
Asiago cheese bagel	330	6	3.5
Cinnamon crunch bagel	430	8	5
Cinnamon swirl bagel	320	2.5	1
Dutch apple & raisin bagel	360	3	1
Everything bagel	300	2.5	0
Plain bagel	290	1.5	0
Sesame bagel	310	3	0
French toast bagel	350	5	2
Whole grain bagel	370	3.5	0
Pecan braid pastry	440	25	11
Carrot walnut muffin	430	19	4

Sodium (mg)	Carbs (g)	Fiber (g)	Sugar (g)
890	12	3	5
60	31	2	25
290	76	1	63
130	73	0	63
140	72	0	54
170	32	3	13
370	66	3	32
570	55	2	3
430	81	3	30
460	65	3	11
620	77	2	33
630	59	2	4
450	59	2	3
450	59	2	3
610	67	2	15
420	70	6	5
270	46	2	20
380	61	2	33

Panera Bread	Cals	Fat (g)	SatFat (g)
BREAKFAST			
Reduced fat wild blueberry muffin	360	10	2
Wild blueberry muffin	390	15	2.5
Wild blueberry scone	390	16	11
Cinnamon roll	620	24	14
Pecan roll	720	38	11
Spinach/artichoke baked egg soufflé	500	32	18
Spinach/bacon baked egg soufflé	570	37	20
Turkey/sausage/ potato baked egg soufflé	460	28	15
Bacon/egg/cheese grilled breakfast sandwich	510	24	10
Sausage/egg/cheese grilled breakfast sandwich	550	30	12
SANDWICHES			
Half chicken bacon Dijon on Country	470	18	7
Half chicken bacon Dijon on French	390	18	7
Half Smokehouse turkey on Focaccia	430	18	6
Half Smokehouse turkey on Three Cheese	410	15	7
Half tomato & mozzarella on ciabatta	390	15	5

Sodium (mg)	Carbs (g)	Fiber (g)	Sugar (g)
220	61	1	35
290	58	1	34
780	56	2	23
480	89	3	33
310	88	2	48
830	35	2	6
990	36	2	6
600	35	2	6
1060	44	2	2
800	44	2	2
1010	48	2	7
770	32	1	8
1310	41	2	4
1330	41	2	3
650	50	4	5

Panera Bread	Cals	Fat (g)	SatFat (g)
SANDWICHES			
Half turkey artichoke on focaccia	370	13	3.5
Half Asiago roast beef on Asiago cheese	360	16	6
Half bacon turkey bravo on tomato basil	420	16	5
Half chipotle chicken on Artisan French	530	28	7
Half Italian combo on ciabatta	520	23	9
Half chicken salad on sesame semolina	360	13	2.5
Half chicken salad on whole grain	320	13	2.5
Half smoked ham & Swiss on rye	350	18	7
Half smoked ham & Swiss on stone-milled rye	390	14	5
Half smoked turkey breast on Country	310	9	1.5
Half smoked turkey breast on sourdough	240	9	1.5
Half tuna salad on honey wheat	380	23	4.5
SALADS			
Baked potato soup, 8 oz (You Pick Two size)	230	14	9
Broccoli cheddar soup, 8 oz (You Pick Two size)	190	10	6

Sodium (mg)	Carbs (g)	Fiber (g)	Sugar (g)
1170	44	3	5
640	29	1	2
1460	43	2	4
1280	43	2	3
1530	47	2	3
970	50	7	5
770	40	9	5
940	28	2	4
1290	41	3	3
1040	40	2	2
840	25	1	2
570	32	3	6
720	21	2	3
1020	16	5	0

Panera Bread	Cals	Fat (g)	SatFat (g)
SALADS			
Cream of chicken/wild rice (You Pick Two size)	200	12	6
Creamy tomato (You Pick Two size)	210	15	8
French onion w/cheese & Croutons (You Pick Two size)	90	3	1.5
Low-fat chicken noodle (You Pick Two size)	100	2	0
New England clam chowder (You Pick Two size)	450	34	20

Starbucks			
COLD DRINKS			
Blended strawberry lemonade, tall	200	0	0
Caffe vanilla Frappuccino w/o whip, tall	230	2.5	1.5
Caffe vanilla Frappuccino w/whip, tall	320	10	6
Caramel Frappuccino blended coffee w/o whip, tall	220	3	2
Caramel Frappuccino blended coffee w/whip, tall	300	11	7

Sodium (mg)	Carbs (g)	Fiber (g)	Sugar (g)
970	19	1	2
770	20	3	10
1560	13	1	4
1110	16	1	1
1190	29	3	0
0	49	1	47
180	49	0	43
190	52	0	45
180	44	0	38
190	46	0	39

Starbucks	Cals	Fat (g)	SatFat (g)
COLD DRINKS			
Caramel Frappuccino light blended coffee, tall	130	1	0
Cinnamon Dolce Frappuccino blended coffee w/whip, tall	290	10	6
Cinnamon Dolce Frappuccino light blended coffee, tall	120	0.5	0
Coffee Frappuccino blended coffee, tall	120	2.5	1.5
Coffee Frappuccino light blended coffee, tall	90	0.5	0
Espresso Frappuccino blended coffee, tall	140	1.5	1
Espresso Frappuccino light blended coffee, tall	80	0	0
Iced apple Chai infusion, tall	170	0	0
Iced brewed coffee, tall	60	0	0
Iced caffe Americano, tall	10	0	0
Iced caffe latte w/2% milk, tall	100	3.5	2.5
Iced caffe mocha w/2% milk, whip, tall	230	12	7
Iced caffe mocha w/2% milk w/o whip, tall	150	4.5	2
Iced Tazo green latte w/2% milk, tall	190	4	2.5

Sodium (mg)	Carbs (g)	Fiber (g)	Sugar (g)
180	25	2	18
190	45	0	39
180	24	2	17
170	37	0	31
160	18	2	12
125	27	0	22
140	16	2	10
10	44	0	40
0	15	0	15
5	2	0	0
80	10	0	9
70	29	1	21
60	26	1	20
85	31	1	30

Starbucks	Cals	Fat (g)	SatFat (g)
COLD DRINKS			
Iced vanilla latte w/2% milk, tall	140	3	2
Java chip Frappuccino light blended coffee, tall	160	3.5	2
Mocha Frappuccino blended coffee w/o whip, tall	200	3	1.5
Mocha Frappuccino blended coffee w/whip, tall	280	11	6
Mocha Frappuccino light blended coffee, tall	110	1	0
Tazo black shaken iced tea, tall	60	0	0
Tazo black shaken iced tea lemonade, tall	100	0	0
Tazo Chai Frappuccino blended crème w/o whip, tall	260	1.5	0
Tazo Chai Frappuccino blended crème w/whip, tall	340	10	5
Tazo Chai iced tea latte w/2% milk, tall	180	3	2
Tazo green shaken iced tea, tall	60	0	0
Tazo green shaken iced tea lemonade, tall	100	0	0
HOT DRINKS			
Caffe Americano w/2% milk, tall	10	0	0

Sodium (mg)	Carbs (g)	Fiber (g)	Sugar (g)
70	23	0	21
180	30	3	20
170	41	0	34
180	43	0	36
170	23	2	15
10	16	0	15
10	25	0	25
220	52	0	44
230	55	0	45
70	33	0	31
10	16	0	15
10	25	0	25
5	2	0	0

Starbucks	Cals	Fat (g)	SatFat (g)
HOT DRINKS			
Caffe latte w/2% milk, tall	150	6	3.5
Caffe mocha w/2% milk w/o whip, tall	200	6	3.5
Caffe mocha w/2% milk w/whip, tall	270	12	7
Cappuccino w/2% milk, tall	90	3.5	2
Caramel Macchiato w/2% milk, tall	180	5	3.5
Cinnamon Dolce crème w/2% milk, w/o whip, tall	210	6	3.5
Cinnamon Dolce crème w/2% milk, w/whip, tall	270	12	7
Cinnamon Dolce latte w/2% milk, w/o whip, tall	200	5	3
Coffee of the week, tall	5	0	0
Decaf coffee of the week, tall	5	0	0
Espresso truffle w/o whip, tall	300	9	5
Espresso truffle w/whip, tall	360	15	9
Gingersnap latte w/2% milk, w/o whip, tall	210	5	3
BREAKFAST			
Butter croissant	310	18	11
Multigrain bagel	320	4	0
Plain bagel	300	1	0

Sodium (mg)	Carbs (g)	Fiber (g)	Sugar (g)
115	14	0	13
100	31	1	24
105	33	1	26
70	9	0	8
100	25	0	23
120	31	0	31
125	32	0	32
110	30	0	29
10	0	0	0
10	0	0	0
110	43	5	3
115	45	5	31
110	31	0	27
290	32	trace	4
220	62	4	8
460	64	2	8

Starbucks	Cals	Fat (g)	SatFat (g)
BREAKFAST			
Morning bun	350	16	9
Blueberry streusel muffin	360	11	6
Perfect oatmeal	140	2.5	0.5
Perfect oatmeal topping: brown sugar	50	0	0
Perfect oatmeal topping: dried fruit	100	0	0
Perfect oatmeal topping: nut medley	100	9	1
Bacon, gouda cheese, egg frittata on artisan roll	380	20	8
Classic sausage, egg & aged cheddar sandwich	500	29	9
Ham, egg frittata, cheddar cheese on artisan roll	370	16	6
Reduced-fat egg white turkey bacon sandwich	340	10	3
SALADS			
Chop Chop pasta salad	480	26	8
Farmers Market salad w/dressing	300	20	5
Fruit & cheese plate	380	21	11
DESSERTS			
Black & white cookies, 2	240	12	1

Sodium (mg)	Carbs (g)	Fiber (g)	Sugar (g)
330	45	2	19
390	59	2	33
105	25	4	0
0	13	0	13
10	24	2	20
0	2	1	1
1050	31	0	1
980	42	2	3
730	32	0	1
750	47	3	6
1340	32	2	2
350	24	4	16
530	37	3	24
160	32	1	22

Starbucks	Cals	Fat (g)	SatFat (g)
DESSERTS			
Outrageous oatmeal cookie	370	14	8
Banana nut bread	480	19	2.5
Marble loaf	330	12	5
Blueberry scone	500	23	13
Cinnamon chip scone	470	18	10
Maple oat pecan scone	470	21	11

Sodium (mg)	Carbs (g)	Fiber (g)	Sugar (g)
170	56	3	36
210	73	4	44
480	50	1	32
640	68	2	21
390	63	2	26
270	64	5	16

CHAPTER SEVEN

Heart-Healthy Supplements from A to Z

If you already take some form of nutritional supplements—vitamins, minerals, proteins, fiber, herbs (sometimes referred to as "botanicals") or other substances—you have plenty of company. The National Institutes of Health (NIH) says 52 percent of American adults take these over-the-counter tablets, powders, capsules or liquids to boost our health; in Britain that figure jumps to nearly 60 percent, and among elderly Americans it's a mighty 72 percent. In this country alone, supplements are a $20 billion business.

There is a growing body of scientific evidence that some nutritional supplements can improve cholesterol levels, even as a natural alternative to statin medications. Only you and your doctor can decide when that choice might be appropriate. Because supplementation is an option in building a heart-healthy life, we're presenting it here, with recommendations for using each supplement.

WHY TAKE SUPPLEMENTS?

People supplement their diets, of course, because they want to be healthy and they believe that taking supplements will help them accomplish that. It's always best to get your nutrients from food, if possible, and Chapter 4 gave you a rundown on healthy fats, carbohydrates, fiber sources, and other nutrients you need in a heart-healthy diet. In Chapter 5, you read about bringing together the best food choices for your own diet, and how TLC (Therapeutic Lifestyle Change) can give you a template for creating an eating plan you can stick with and enjoy for life.

As a layperson, it can be difficult to know which supplement is right for you. Like so many health-related products, nutritional supplements often are marketed with a lot of hype—who can sort through the sales pitches and confusion? So we did the research for you. This chapter presents nutritional supplements that have been found, in rigorous scientific studies, to influence cholesterol levels in a healthy way. Many people working to manage their cholesterol levels try one or two of these supplements; we've presented a long list simply to give you more choices. If you aim to lower your cholesterol level and enhance your heart health, you may want to consider incorporating natural supplements into your new TLC plan.

SAFETY WITH SUPPLEMENTS

Because dietary supplements are classified as foods, rather than drugs, the U.S. government's restrictions on them are not as rigid. While selecting any supplement, it's important to keep the following pointers in mind.

- Unlike medications, companies that manufacture supplements don't have to prove their safety or effectiveness before you buy them—yet they can make health claims if any research findings exist to support their claims. What this means for you: Buy supplements *only* produced by established, respected manufacturers.

- Once a supplement is on the market, the U.S. Food and Drug Administration (FDA) does monitor its safety, and the Federal Trade Commission (FTC) monitors its advertising.

- Be a detective and protect yourself from possible interactions and other harmful effects of the supplements you've chosen. You'll find an abundance of solid information with The National Center for Complementary and Alternative Medicine (NCCAM) at nccam.nih.gov, and the NIH Office of Dietary Supplements, dietary-supplements.info.nih.gov.

- Tell your physician and pharmacist which supplements you are taking, so they are aware of possible interactions with medications or with each other.

- Check the expiration dates on the packaging. Most dietary supplements are plant- and animal-based substances, and they can spoil. They also can lose their effectiveness or change their composition after they expire, so be sure to buy from a fresh batch.

- Do not take nutritional supplements without talking to your healthcare provider if you're planning to have surgery in the next two months. Some supplements increase your risk of bleeding, or they interact with anesthesia.

- Likewise if you are pregnant, nursing a baby or planning to give the supplement to a child, talk to a health professional before using it. Not all supplements have been tested on pregnant women, nursing mothers or children.

- Read the label! You may not want to ingest all the ingredients in the supplement. Many contain iron, for instance, which isn't a healthy additive for everyone. Herbal supplements can contain many compounds, and you won't know which ingredients are active. Some supplements are best taken with food, others on an empty stomach; some are most effective if you take them before you exercise, while others should be taken at bedtime. Proper storage and dosages are important as well—all information you will find on the label.

- Finally, cholesterol isn't the only "condition" that will be affected by your supplement choice—another good reason to first talk with your doctor or pharmacist. If you are on a low-calorie diet, you may also need certain vitamins added. If you are lactose-intolerant, you may need to supplement with calcium, and women taking birth control or estrogen replacement probably need folic acid and vitamin B_6.

GOOD-CHOLESTEROL SUPPLEMENTS

Now that you have a solid awareness of supplements in general, you can begin selecting one or more that can enhance your feeling of well-being and help keep your cholesterol levels in check.

On the following pages, we've provided information on twenty-four nutritional supplements that have demonstrated a healthy effect on cholesterol levels in scientific studies. Each supplement's write-up is divided into four sections.

- *Background.* This is the lowdown for this individual supplement, an introductory paragraph or two on its history, its other roles, and more interesting information.
- *Heart-healthy effects.* Here we share what we know about the supplement's positive effects on cholesterol.
- *How to use it.* If a specific dosage or form is recommended for this supplement, this is where you'll find it.
- *Cautions, side effects.* Beyond common sense, we offer tips for using supplements safely and alert you to known possible risks.

We've listed the supplements in alphabetical order. To simplify your search for the best supplement(s) for *you*, the most popular and proven cholesterol-lowering supplements are marked with an asterisk (*).

ARTICHOKE LEAF EXTRACT

Produced from dried artichoke leaves, this extract, also known as *Cynara scolymus*, is an antioxidant-packed "liver tonic" that helps digestion and nausea. It contains cynarin, a substance that increases the liver's bile production and causes it to flow more quickly from the gallbladder, thus possibly helping us excrete more cholesterol. (Bile aids in digesting fats.) Artichoke also may limit the synthesis of cholesterol in our bodies.

Heart-healthy Effects

In 2000, a group of 150 adults with high-risk cholesterol levels participated in a German study; half of them took 1,800 mg of artichoke leaf extract per day for six weeks and the other half took a placebo. The results were impressive: Those taking artichoke leaf lowered their total cholesterol by 18.5 percent, compared to the placebo group's 8.6 percent. Moreover, the artichoke leaf group lowered their LDL cholesterol by 22.9 percent and the placebo group lowered theirs by just 6 percent. Smaller studies have since supported those findings, but the evidence remains scant. Still, the Mayo Clinic is among those institutions that agree artichoke leaf extract could help lower both LDL and total cholesterol.

How to Use It

To help reduce cholesterol levels, 1,200 mg to 1,800 mg per day are recommended, divided into two or three doses.

Your best bet for getting an exact dose is to purchase artichoke leaf tablets at a health food store. You also can find fresh or dried artichoke leaves (for making a tea or tincture) at some health food stores, as well as juices and liquid extracts. With do-it-yourself methods, however, measuring a correct dose can be nearly impossible, and the liquid forms can leave a bitter taste. (And no one could eat enough artichokes every day to make a difference in their cholesterol levels.)

Cautions, Side Effects

The only reported side effects are gas and slight nausea. As with any food, however, an allergy is always possible.

BLOND PSYLLIUM

Blond psyllium, or psyllium seed, is a well-known natural laxative that also can help lower cholesterol levels. It's high in soluble fiber, which you read in Chapter 4 is an important weapon in combating unhealthy cholesterol; psyllium is so high in fiber, in fact, that it could double as a fiber supplement. In its natural form, it is a non-wheat grain, coated with a sticky substance that, when mixed into water, becomes gummy. The body can't digest this gummy matter; instead it sticks to cholesterol coming into the body from food.

Heart-healthy Effects

When the gummy matter from blond psyllium attaches itself to cholesterol from our food, it is eliminated with food waste—along with the cholesterol—because we cannot digest it. By that elimination, it lowers our cholesterol levels. Psyllium also carries the added benefits of helping to lower blood sugar.

How to Use It

Health food stores sell already-prepared psyllium seed powder, though many such preparations contain added sugar; if you choose a prepared powder, check the label for added ingredients. You also can buy seed husks, which you would grind yourself. The recommended dosage varies with the source, ranging from 2,500 mg to five grams, mixed with a full glass of water, twice a day. We recommend talking to your physician and starting with a lower dose.

Or, you can take the easier route and use a commercial fiber product such as Metamucil, which contains blond psyllium. Follow the directions on the label.

Cautions, Side Effects

Blond psyllium can cause stomach pain, diarrhea, constipation and nausea, so it's important to talk with your doctor before using it.

CALCIUM*

We're guessing every reader is familiar with this one—but probably not as a cholesterol-lowering supplement. You know calcium as a bone-strengthener, and studies now suggest it may improve cholesterol as well by increasing our HDL cholesterol levels.

Calcium is our bodies' most plentiful mineral. While 99 percent of our calcium is stored in our bones and teeth, the other 1 percent is critical for a number of functions; only with calcium can we contract our muscles, transmit impulses throughout our nervous systems, and be confident that our blood vessels are expanding and contracting as needed.

Heart-healthy Effects

In recent years, scientists also have begun affirming that calcium may help cholesterol levels. They noticed for years that people living in areas with "hard" water had less heart disease than those who drank soft water; studies show that total cholesterol can be lowered by up to 4 percent by taking

1,000 mg of calcium daily. Looking at HDL and LDL separately, some studies showed that the same amount of elemental calcium—that is, the amount of calcium available for absorption from that dose—can raise HDL by between 1 and 5 percent and lower LDL by 2 to 6 percent. But you should note, too, that a number of studies showed no change in HDL and LDL cholesterol levels at all.

In light of that disparity in findings, current wisdom says that if you need to lower your cholesterol, calcium alone isn't the best choice—but because it brings such major benefits for bone health (especially for postmenopausal women), supplementing with calcium still is highly recommended.

How to Use It

When you read the label on a jar of calcium supplements, look for a term mentioned above—"elemental calcium." It refers to the amount of actual calcium that will be absorbed from that dose, rather than the weight of the pills, and it is the most important phrase on the label. You may see other types of calcium lingo, such as calcium citrate, calcium lactate or calcium gluconate—all terms referring to the substances to which the calcium binds, not the amount of calcium you'll actually absorb into your system. For instance, 500 mg of calcium carbonate only contains 200 mg of elemental calcium, so instead of getting 500 mg of calcium if you take that pill, you'll only be getting 200 mg.

As for the best dosage, that depends on your age. During the formative years (ages nine to eighteen), you should get 1,300 mg/day. From nineteen to fifty, the optimal dose is 1,000 mg, and after age fifty, you should get 1,200 mg/day—and remember, those dosages refer to *elemental* calcium. A good way to remember which type of calcium you should count: It's *elementary*, my dear! And always take that 1,200 mg of calcium with 400 IU of vitamin D so the calcium will be absorbed into your system.

Cautions, Side Effects

Taking more calcium than you need can lead to constipation, bloating and gas, so take only the recommended dose for your age. If you have chronic kidney disease, kidney stones, prostate cancer or hyperparathyroidism, be sure to talk with a doctor before taking calcium supplements or you could aggravate your symptoms. And if you take calcium long-term, some research suggests it may compete with other minerals for absorption, so consider taking a vitamin/mineral supplement—again after talking it over with your doctor.

CARNITINE*

Technically a B-vitamin, L-Carnitine, its most commonly seen form, is similar to B-complex vitamins in its water solubility and the fact that it can be produced by the liver. Some individuals don't produce enough carnitine, while others don't metabolize it efficiently.

Small amounts of carnitine are found in a host of everyday foods, including almonds, artichokes, asparagus, bananas, beans, broccoli, cashews, garlic, oatmeal, soy beans, sunflower seeds, walnuts and whole wheat. It's also found in several herbs, including ginger, horseradish, nettle and sassafras. It's easy to counter carnitine's benefits, however, by drinking alcohol, coffee or tea, or by eating refined sugar.

Heart-healthy Effects

Integrative medicine experts have known for years that carnitine helps us to utilize dietary fats and fatty acids; in burning fatty acids, carnitine helps to lower LDL cholesterol and triglyceride levels, and raise HDL levels. It also helps to regulate blood sugar and, by assisting muscles during exercise, helps us to burn fat and lose weight.

How to Use It

Manufacturers of L-carnitine vary widely in their recommended dosages. Taking 500 mg daily is generally considered safe, but talk with your doctor before starting on this supplement.

Cautions, Side Effects

The most common side effect of L-carnitine is nervous energy; it can lead to insomnia or even a rapid heartbeat. People on thyroid medications should avoid L-carnitine unless they have a doctor's go-ahead because this supplement can interfere with the medicine and diminish its effectiveness. Do not take L-carnitine (or other supplements) if you are on kidney dialysis.

CHITOSAN

Derived from the hard shells of crustaceans (think shrimp and crabs), chitosan supplements have been on health-food store shelves for years, sold as a "fat attractor" that may facilitate weight loss. However, scientific studies testing chitosan's performance as a fat blocker have produced mixed results, and the FDA has issued letters to several companies that make unproven claims regarding the supplement's weight-loss capabilities.

Heart-healthy Effects

That said, obese individuals in one study who took chitosan and followed a low-calorie diet lowered their total cholesterol levels by 25 percent. But since weight loss can lower cholesterol levels significantly, researchers couldn't be certain whether the lower levels were due to chitosan or weight loss.

Participants in another study lowered their total cholesterol by 6 percent and raised their HDL by 7 percent. Others studies suggested chitosan may not affect cholesterol levels at all.

How to Use It

Because of the conflicting research, it's probably not wise to rely exclusively on chitosan for lowering your cholesterol.

Cautions, Side Effects

Because chitosan may block some fat absorption, it also may block absorption of fat-soluble vitamins (A, D, E and K) and some minerals. If you decide to take it to help lose weight, supplement also with a good multivitamin and consult your doctor to make sure it won't interact with any of your medications. You also may experience flatulence, bloating, diarrhea, constipation and fatty stools.

CINNAMON

You stir cinnamon into coffee and sprinkle it on your oatmeal. Who knew it also is good for you?

Cinnamon is harvested from the bark of the evergreen cinnamon tree that grows in the tropics. It contains high-powered antioxidants that make cinnamon a terrific anti-aging, anti-free radical garnish.

Heart-healthy Effects

In the most widely-quoted study of cinnamon's healthy effects, published in *Diabetes Care*, participants' total cholesterol levels were reduced by 12 to 26 percent, and their LDL was lowered 7 to 27 percent, depending on which study subgroup they belonged to. While their HDL was barely raised, their triglycerides were reduced by 23 to 30 percent. What's more, they lowered their glucose levels by 18 to 29 percent.

How to Use It

In recipes you may want to follow directions, but for casual cinnamon use, a "healthy sprinkle" works well. It doesn't take much to get the healthy effects; half a teaspoon daily can reduce blood sugar by 25 percent. For a fresher taste, buy cinnamon sticks instead of already-ground and use a grater to add sprinkles to your food. Cinnamon sticks also are a terrific aid when you need an "oral fix," such as when you're trying to stop smoking cigarettes. Just suck on them; one stick will last for hours.

Cautions, Side Effects

As far as we know, cinnamon doesn't interact with any medications. If you're allergic to cinnamon, it could cause a rash or bronchial constriction, but such side effects are rare. Pregnant women should avoid cinnamon bark and cinnamon oil.

COENZYME Q_{10}*

Our bodies produce coenzyme Q_{10}, in the mitochondria—or stringy, tubelike mini-sections—of every cell. It helps produce the cells' energy source, a substance called ATP, and is a powerful antioxidant. As we age, though, our coenzyme Q_{10} levels diminish; people with heart disease, cancer and diabetes often have low coenzyme Q_{10}.

Heart-healthy Benefits

Some studies show that coenzyme Q_{10} helps reduce leg swelling and could have a positive effect on high blood pressure. It might also be good for treating headaches, fibromyalgia and symptoms of congestive heart failure. There also is evidence that people who take coenzyme Q_{10} within three days following a heart attack have a smaller chance of suffering another heart attack or chest pains.

For those already taking statin drugs to lower their cholesterol, coenzyme Q_{10} may deter muscle-related discomfort sometimes associated with such medicines. It's easy to see why coenzyme Q_{10} is such a popular supplement for people experiencing any variety of heart problems!

How to Use It

Readily available at any pharmacy, coenzyme Q_{10} is available in pills and as a mouth spray. The usual dose is 100 to 200 mg daily—but for those with high blood pressure, congestive heart failure or who've experienced a heart attack, your doctor may recommend a different dose. Take it with a meal containing some fat so it will be absorbed. Some experts also recommend coenzyme Q_{10} for women who have been treated for breast cancer; the evidence is scant, but several studies have found it might help prevent the cancer from recurring or spreading.

Cautions, Side Effects

Mild, possible side effects can include nausea, vomiting, diarrhea, rash, headache, dizziness, insomnia, appetite loss and irritability. Coenzyme Q_{10} can lower blood sugar, so if you have diabetes or hypoglycemia, or take medications or supplements that affect blood sugar, talk to your doctor before taking coenzyme Q_{10}.

Little is known about the effects of coenzyme Q_{10} on women who are pregnant or breastfeeding, so it's best to avoid taking it during those times.

CHROMIUM

For a trace mineral, chromium has a big job: It's an essential part of a substance called glucose tolerance factor (GTF), which works to keep our blood glucose levels balanced. It occurs naturally in eggs, liver, onions, potatoes, tomatoes, whole grains, beer and wine, but processing foods may reduce the amount of chromium in them—and therefore eating too many processed foods can lead to a chromium deficiency and, consequently, insulin resistance.

Heart-healthy Effects

Some studies have shown that chromium can help lower high cholesterol levels, thereby lowering the risk of heart disease.

How to Use It

Although it's available at virtually every drugstore, chromium can be a confusing purchase because of its many forms—chromium picolinate, chromium polynicotinate, chromium chloride and chromium-enriched yeast.

The most popular form is chromium picolinate because it's the most easily absorbed into our systems. (Supplementing with 200 to 400 mcg per day is recommended.) However, people with diabetes may prefer chromium polynicotinate because it contains vitamin B_3, or niacin (profiled later in this chapter), a natural blood-sugar stabilizer.

Cautions, Side Effects

Women who are pregnant or breastfeeding may need a higher-than-usual dose. Also, if you are supplementing with both chromium and calcium carbonate, be aware that the calcium will counteract the chromium and interfere with its dosage. Talk to your healthcare provider if this is a concern.

FISH OIL*

Those who advocate taking nutritional supplements don't always agree with the medical establishment, but when it comes to fish oil, they heartily agree: If you are at risk for coronary disease, take fish oil.

The name means, literally, oil found in fish—not actually an oil produced by their bodies, but omega-3 fatty acids from the algae and plankton the fish eat. The two best-known omega-3s are EPA (eicosapentaenoic acid) and DHA (docosahexaenoic acid).

Heart-healthy benefits

One of the highest-recommended supplements for heart health, fish oil has been proven in study after study to lower cholesterol and, in larger doses, triglycerides. It is an anti-inflammatory agent that also lowers blood pressure, can prevent death after a heart attack, thins the blood slightly, and can help regulate your heartbeat. Importantly, it also can convert small, dense LDL into the fluffier, less harmful type.

The Cardiovascular Health Study concluded that the higher the level of omega-3 fatty acids, the lower your risk of a fatal heart attack. The evidence is especially strong in reducing the death rate for men who have suffered heart attacks.

How to Use It

First, buy fish oil capsules that were produced by a reliable supplement manufacturer, and check the expiration date on the bottle. Poor-quality fish oil will turn rancid and give off a fish-garbage smell—and leave a fishy aftertaste. When you get the capsules home, break one open to be sure you have a fresh batch.

The usual dose is 1 to 4 grams per day, with the higher dosage for people who need to lower their triglycerides.

Cautions, Side Effects

People taking blood thinning medications such as warfarin (Coumadin) should talk to a doctor before taking fish oil capsules, as there may be an interaction. Pregnant or breast-feeding women, or people with diabetes, also should consult a doctor before using fish oil. If you have a seafood allergy, don't take fish oil. The supplement also can cause bad breath, gas, nausea, vomiting or diarrhea.

FLAXSEED

Culled from the flax plant, flaxseeds are tiny, shiny seeds used by the ancient Greeks and Romans for both cooking and medicine. They're packed with ALA (alpha-linolenic acid), an omega-3 fatty acid, along with a high fiber content and lignan, an antioxidant and phytoestrogen, or estrogenlike plant material, that also contains fiber.

Heart-healthy effects

Research has shown that adding flax to your diet lowers your total cholesterol by as much as 9 percent over four weeks, and your LDL by up to 18 percent. Flaxseed also may reduce triglycerides and can help maintain a healthy blood pressure and blood sugar level.

How to use it

Add a tablespoon or two to your daily food by sprinkling it over cereal or hot veggies, adding it to soup or homemade bread, or stirring it into a smoothie. For freshness and maximum nutrition, buy flaxseeds whole and grind them each day.

Cautions, side effects

Flaxseed can interact with blood thinners such as aspirin, warfarin (Coumadin) or clopidogrel (Plavix), so people taking these medications should talk with a healthcare provider before taking flaxseed. It also can cause bloating, gas or diarrhea.

GARLIC

You use it to flavor hundreds of dishes, and no doubt your parents counseled you to chew a little if you had the flu. Louis Pasteur discovered garlic's ability to fight bacteria in 1858, and natural health enthusiasts have been promoting its healing powers ever since. People either love garlic or hate it, for the same reason—its organosulfur compounds, the substances that create its sharp taste and smell.

Heart-healthy Effects

There's good news and bad news about taking garlic for heart health: The Agency for Healthcare Research and Quality did report in 2000 that garlic caused a small drop in total cholesterol and LDL. The bad news then was, the cholesterol-lowering benefit lasted for only three months. Later research by the Archives of Internal Medicine showed no effect on cholesterol or triglycerides at all, while another 2007 study found that garlic did lower LDL and total cholesterol slightly.

How to use it

If you choose to take your garlic raw, one to two cloves daily will provide the health benefits. Or, you can mince it and stir it into a tomato sauce, or slice it and spread it on whole-grain bread. You also can take a 300 mg garlic capsule to bypass the taste and smell.

Cautions, Side Effects

Garlic interferes with blood's clotting ability and interacts with blood thinners, so eat a minimal amount if you're already taking a blood-thinning medication. It also can cause nausea, heartburn, gas, diarrhea, or perhaps the biggest reasons why many people avoid it—bad breath and body odor.

GREEN TEA

This beverage is so good for you it almost rivals broccoli, and some archaeologists believe we've been sipping green tea for up to 500,000 years. It's been used by Indian and Chinese healers for generations, believed to enhance heart health, give us energy, heal wounds and help us to focus. It's richer in polyphenols (powerful antioxidants) than black tea or oolong tea.

Heart-healthy Effects

Studies show that the primary polyphenol in green tea, EGCG (epigallocatechin gallate), has anti-inflammatory qualities, giving green tea the ability to help lower total cholesterol and LDL, and raise HDL cholesterol. It also reduces inflammation associated with some other conditions, including Crohn's disease, and may help prevent skin tumors and obesity.

How to Use It

Just two to three cups of green tea per day will bestow its health benefits. If you're not a tea drinker, you can buy green tea extract in capsules; the standard dose is 300 to 400 mg daily. Read the label; you'll want capsules containing at least 70 percent of polyphenols per dose.

Cautions, side effects

If you are sensitive to caffeine, be aware that one green tea-bag typically contains 20 mg of caffeine—much less than the same amount of black tea (40 mg), cola (45 mg) or coffee (80 mg), but it may be enough to affect you. Also, pregnant women should keep in mind that EGCG affects our ability to fully use folate, which helps prevent birth defects in newborns. Research hasn't given a clear answer as to how much green tea you'd have to drink in order for your folate to be affected by it, but many women stop drinking green tea until after they give birth for that reason.

KRILL OIL

Sometimes confused with fish oil, krill oil is produced from Antarctic crustaceans similar to shrimp. Like fish oil, krill oil contains EPA and DHA, but also antioxidants (such as astaxanthin, powerful in the fight against free radicals) and phospholipids, which we need for building cell membranes.

Heart-healthy Effects

If your aim is to lower your triglycerides, then some experts recommend fish oil, with its higher concentrations of EPA and DHA, over krill oil. But a twelve-week Canadian study concluded that krill oil did better at reducing LDL by 34 percent while also increasing HDL cholesterol by 4.2 percent.

It also may be effective at reducing symptoms of arthritis and premenstrual syndrome (PMS).

How to Use It

Capsules are the easiest way to supplement with krill oil. A dose of 500 mg daily is the usual recommendation; some experts advise taking up to 1,000 mg.

Cautions, Side Effects

Krill oil can cause diarrhea, loose stools or indigestion. It won't become rancid and leave a fishy aftertaste, but don't take it if you have a seafood allergy or bleeding disorder.

MAGNESIUM*

Favored for years as a supplement to enhance bone health, magnesium now is known to also reduce LDL cholesterol and raise HDL cholesterol.

About 65 percent of our body's magnesium lives in our bones, so the connection to strong bones is understandable. It also helps metabolize fats and carbohydrates, helps build protein and helps reduce metabolic syndrome—a collection of disorders that include low HDL and high triglyceride levels—among other benefits.

Heart-healthy Effects

In addition to lowering LDL and raising HDL levels, magnesium impacts heart health by helping to lower blood pressure, assisting the body in ridding itself of excess sodium through the kidneys and, indirectly, helping people with type 2 diabetes to regulate their blood sugar levels.

How to Use It

The FDA recommends 420 mg for men and 320 mg for women over age thirty. Pregnant women may need more, but speak to your doctor before taking a higher amount.

Cautions, Side Effects

Taking excess amounts of magnesium could cause drowsiness or diarrhea, while a deficiency could play a part in PMS, high blood pressure, insomnia, constipation and kidney stones. It's best to talk to your healthcare practitioner before taking them.

NIACIN*

You may know it as vitamin B_3; technically it's called nicotinic acid. Niacin's primary job is to convert carbohydrates into energy. It also plays a key role in keeping your skin, hair, eyes, and nervous and digestive systems at their best.

You'll find niacin included in most multivitamins, but it's also sold separately in higher doses for consumers with a vitamin B_3 deficiency and those who are trying to lower their cholesterol.

Heart-healthy Effects

Niacin is a real cholesterol-lowering performer in a number of studies. It's proven to lower LDL by as much as 25 percent, boost HDL by up to 35 percent, and lower triglycerides by 24 percent—which makes it one of the most effective substances available for battling high cholesterol.

How to Use It

Talk to a doctor before supplementing with niacin because it comes in various forms, and one may be better for you than another—and excess niacin can cause dangerous side effects.

Dosage usually falls between 500 mg and 2,000 mg daily. Doctors sometimes prescribe niacin, either as an over-the-counter supplement or as prescription medication, in addition to statin drugs. One prescription drug, Niaspan, is an extended-release form of niacin, which some people may prefer for the convenience.

Cautions, Side Effects

The most common side effect of niacin is "flushing"—your skin reddens and is warm to the touch. Flushing usually is temporary and can be counteracted by taking niacin with food or aspirin (if taken before you take the niacin). Other possible side effects include headache, dizziness, diarrhea, coughing, skin tingling, itching, liver damage and higher blood sugar.

PYCNOGENOL

This fascinating supplement comes from only one spot on the planet (and one of the loveliest), the Burgundy coast of southwest France. Extracted from the bark of the maritime pine growing there, pycnogenol has proven effective in combating a long list of conditions, from diabetic retinopathy to migraines. (I can personally attest to its effectiveness in combating swollen feet and ankles during long plane rides and long sessions sitting at a desk.) It's one of those ingredients that no one heard of until recently; now it's found in anti-aging creams, an ingredient in some multi-vitamins, and as a stand-alone supplement.

Heart-healthy Effects

Two studies have shown pycnogenol to reduce LDL cholesterol from 7 to 16 percent. The positive effect lasted only while subjects took pycnogenol, and ended when they stopped taking it.

How to Use It

Because of its many other benefits, pycnogenol may be a worthwhile supplement, but it's not recommended as the single solution to a cholesterol problem. Dosage ranges from 100 mg to 360 mg daily. Supplements are available in pills and capsules, and it's listed as an ingredient in hundreds of anti-aging creams, multivitamins and other products.

Cautions, Side Effects

Minor side effects include dizziness, nausea and mouth ulcers in rare instances. Pycnogenol can stimulate the immune system, possibly increasing symptoms of auto-immune diseases. For that reason, people with lupus, rheumatoid arthritis, multiple sclerosis and some thyroid disorders are advised not to take pycnogenol.

RED YEAST RICE*

You're not going to cook up this "rice" and serve it with beans. Red yeast rice has been popular in traditional Chinese medicine for at least a thousand years to aid circulation and diarrhea; in this country its extract is sold in capsule form. It's a powerful supplement—so potent, in fact, that the FDA has deemed it illegal to sell red yeast rice containing more than trace amounts of certain cholesterol-lowering chemicals, or to promote red yeast rice for reducing cholesterol levels. (Note that we do not "promote" the use of any supplement in this book. Our aim is to present information for readers who want to learn more about their options in lowering their cholesterol levels.)

Heart-healthy Effects

Red yeast rice can lower LDL cholesterol by about 25 percent. It is especially favored by patients who may not want to take a prescription drug because their cholesterol is elevated but not severe. Many practitioners recommend it for patients trying to avoid the side effects of statins, most notably muscle pain and increased liver enzymes. Some doctors practicing alternative medicine prescribe red yeast rice in combination with other substances, such as stanols and sterols.

Most recently, a 2009 study of patients who had stopped taking statin drugs because it caused them muscle pain, lowered their total cholesterol (by 15 percent) and LDL cholesterol (by 21 percent) using red yeast rice.

How to Use It

Red yeast rice is sold in capsules. The usual beginning dose is 600 mg with food, taken twice a day. The maximum is 1,200 mg twice a day.

Cautions, Side Effects

Reported side effects are mile—headaches or stomachache—though heartburn, muscle pain, dizziness, asthma and kidney disease are possible. Women who are pregnant or breastfeeding, and anyone with liver disease or bleeding disorders (or people taking drugs that can increase their risk of bleeding) should not take red yeast rice.

SELENIUM, A CAUTIONARY TALE

Selenium is *not* a cholesterol-lowering supplement—but it's such a popular choice for general health, we decided to include it here as an example of how you actually can *damage* your cholesterol levels by taking supplements in a haphazard way, without doing your research.

A trace essential mineral, selenium is widely known as a powerful antioxidant. But the November 2009 *Journal of Nutrition* published a study by a team at the University of Warwick in which, researchers found that of 1,042 participants, those with high selenium levels also showed an increase in total cholesterol levels of 8 percent, and a 10 percent increase in their LDL cholesterol levels. Interestingly, of those participants with the highest selenium levels, 48.2 percent stated they regularly took dietary supplements.

Although the selenium levels were not caused entirely by supplementing with selenium, the use of selenium supplements had risen sharply in Britain in recent years because of reports that selenium can lower our risk of cancer.

"The cholesterol increases we have identified may have important implications for public health," the lead researcher stated. "In fact, such a difference could translate into a large number of premature deaths from coronary heart disease."

While selenium may have wonderful implications for preventing cancer, this British study is a solid example of the interplay between our physiological systems and the nutrients we take in. It illustrates, in fairly dramatic terms, why we need to talk to a healthcare practitioner before taking any medicine or nutritional supplements.

STANOLS AND STEROLS*

Stanols and sterols are also called phytosterols, or plant sterol and stanol ester, natural compounds found in plant cell membranes. Their molecular structure resembles that of our body's cholesterol, so that when phytosterols enter the body, they compete with cholesterol in our digestive systems—and they win. The cholesterol isn't absorbed, and our cholesterol levels get lower.

Heart-healthy Effects

It's a marvelously effective system. Stanols and sterols can reduce LDL cholesterol levels by as much as 20 percent and total cholesterol by 10 percent, though they have little effect on HDL cholesterol and triglycerides. Still, some experts consider them one of the most effective over-the-counter cholesterol-reducing supplements available.

How to Use It

A daily dose of 2 grams of stanols/sterols can bring about a 10- to 20-percent reduction in LDL cholesterol. Large amounts can be found in certain margarines, but you would have to consume 2 to 4 tablespoons of margarine every day to get the right dosage. In actual food, 1 ounce of almonds contains only 39 mg of phytosterols, so to obtain that daily dose from adding almonds to your diet, you would have to consume more than three pounds of almonds a day! Rye bread, too, contains stanols/sterols—about 33 mg in two slices of bread. To get your daily dose of 2 grams, you would have to consume more loaves than anyone can eat. Obviously, pills are an easier way to supplement with stanols and sterols.

Cautions, Side Effects

Stanols and sterols are well tolerated. Minor side effects can include gas, diarrhea and constipation.

VITAMIN C*

We all know we should load up on vitamin C to keep from catching a cold, and that a healthy dose of vitamin D will help keep our bones stronger as we age. What isn't common knowledge is the role these two vitamins play in maintaining healthy cholesterol levels.

Heart-healthy Effects

Back in 1981, a small study in England found that when elderly patients with vitamin C deficiencies were given 1,000 mg of vitamin C per day, their HDL increased and LDL

lowered somewhat. It was a tenuous finding, since only 11
people participated in the study.

Since then, researchers at the Jean Mayer USDA Human
Nutrition Research Center on Aging at Tufts University
found that taking 1,000 mg of vitamin C daily increased
subjects' HDL cholesterol levels by 7 percent. Their findings
were affirmed by another study, this one done for the National
Institute on Aging in Bethesda, Maryland. That team, which
studied more than 825 men and women between the ages of
nineteen and ninety-five, found that the more vitamin C
their subjects ingested, the higher their HDL cholesterol, to
a maximum of 215 mg of vitamin C daily for women and
346 mg for men. Above those doses, the HDL cholesterol
was no longer affected.

How to Use It

The U.S. Recommended Daily Allowance (RDA) of vitamin C is just 60 mg per day. Most experts agree that up to
250 mg daily is safe and beneficial, and some recommend
up to 1,000 mg.

Cautions, Side Effects

Because vitamin C boosts iron absorption, an excess of vitamin C can invite iron poisoning. Other possible side effects
include diarrhea, indigestion, headaches and fatigue.

VITAMIN D*

Often called the "sunshine vitamin" because our bodies
produce it with short sun exposure, vitamin D usually is
taken to encourage calcium absorption and strong bones.

But scientists also have long known that patients with
diabetes and low levels of vitamin D were at high risk for
heart disease—almost double the general public—and in
2009 they discovered why: Researchers at Washington Uni-

versity School of Medicine in St. Louis found that diabetics with low vitamin D cannot process cholesterol efficiently, so it builds up in their blood vessels—hence the high risk of heart attack and stroke. Supplementing with vitamin D will help those patients.

Heart-healthy Effects

Vitamin D and cholesterol are two sides of the same coin in our bodies: When our systems are operating efficiently, the cholesterol that we produce turns into vitamin D. They appear in the same foods as well; foods that are high in cholesterol also can be high in vitamin D, so that when we switch to a heart-healthy, low-cholesterol diet, we often inadvertently create a vitamin D deficiency.

Vitamin D has proven in many studies to boost HDL cholesterol, while helping to lower LDL cholesterol and triglyceride levels. It's also necessary for bone strength as we age, and supplementing—either alone or with calcium—is a popular choice.

How to Use It

For people with limited sun exposure, or those whose vitamin D levels are low, experts recommend supplements in the form of cholecalciferol (D3), with a daily dose of 1,000 IU.

Cautions, Side Effects

Most adults can tolerate 1,000 IU of vitamin D with no side effects. One caution would be for people taking thiazide diuretic medication; combining it with vitamin D could result in an excess of calcium in the blood.

CHAPTER EIGHT

Lowering Cholesterol with Exercise and a
Balanced Life

Complete TLC includes physical exercise—that sounds like
a chore, but it really isn't!

You can get the exercise you need in a variety of ways,
and you don't have to set aside a lot of time for it. Doing a
little at a time is perfectly acceptable and effective; if you
can't find much time for exercise, do ten or fifteen minutes
at a time. We talk more specifically about what you can do
in the next section.

The point is, regardless of your cholesterol levels and
other health challenges, everyone needs exercise in order to
be strong, energetic and limber, and relaxation in order to
heal, physically and emotionally. You also need relaxation
for heart health, and in this chapter we'll also talk about
some great ways to slow down, calm your anxieties, and
lower your stress level if needed.

EXERCISE: THE BEST MEDICINE

The first thing you need to know: if you are overweight, exercising for weight loss is the single most effective step you
can take for raising your HDL cholesterol, apart from medication intervention. Experts debate all the time as to whether

exercise is more important than diet, but they all agree it's necessary. Can't get around that one.

But look at the control you have over your exercise routine! You alone will decide which exercises are best for you, how frequently you will exercise, how much time you'll spend with it, and whether you will exercise alone or with others.

Regardless of the particulars, TLC lists benefits of regular physical activity for everyone, in addition to healthier cholesterol levels.

- Exercise gives your heart a workout, so it's good for that muscle.

- Active people find it easier to control their weight. Exercisers not only lose more weight than sedentary people, they also maintain their new weight longer.

- One healthy behavior "feeds" another: When you are physically active, you'll discover that it's easier to eat healthier meals, relax with abandon and sleep better at night.

- You will feel better all the time, not just while you're working out.

- You will look more attractive.

- You'll have more choices in clothes (a shopping opportunity!).

- You will feel more confident in all you attempt.

- If you're sluggish now during the day, you really *will* have more energy. Exercise boosts your metabolic rate, so you will burn more calories for hours, not just while you're exercising.

• Gradually, you will become more agile and flexible. If you feel aches and pains daily, that will improve as you become more active and build muscle.

• Exercise can lower your risk of developing colds, respiratory infections, diabetes and even some cancers.

• Physical activity can help relieve stress and anxiety, and boost your mental alertness and memory.

• People who exercise can eat more!

• It's fun to be an active person!

We've known for a long time that even light or moderate exercise can lower your risk of heart disease. A study of 44,500 men in the 1990s, published in the *Journal of the American Medical Association,* found that even half an hour of weight-training per week lowered their risk of heart attacks by 23 percent; even walking briskly for thirty minutes per day lowered their risk by 18 percent. Those who exercised more vigorously but not at length, running a minimum of one hour a week, experienced a whopping 42 percent fewer heart attacks.

Women, too, show remarkable improvement in their heart health when they exercise. A recent study of some 8,700 men and women called the Atherosclerosis Risk in Communities (ARIC) Study, published in 2009 in the *Journal of Lipid Research*, found that over 12 years, both men and women who exercised at least 30 minutes per week doing moderate activities lowered their triglyceride levels and elevated their HDL cholesterol. Only women, however, lowered their LDL cholesterol significantly, with the largest effects found among African American and menopausal women. The fact that any effect at all was found after doing so little activity—only 30 minutes a week—is remarkable.

Even one exercise session can help. Do you sometimes feel, after you've stuffed yourself at a big family dinner, that you should get up and walk around the block? Research shows that you should do just that: Eating a meal high in fat can put fatty deposits in your arteries and restrict blood flow there for up to six hours. Taking that brisk walk can help your arterial function and keep the blood flowing.

There is another side to the exercise coin, however: once you start, you can't stop, at least not without consequences. One study found that increases in HDL and drops in triglyceride levels experienced while the individuals maintained an exercise regimen, reversed themselves once the people stopped exercising. In another study, researchers found that it took just three weeks for people to "lose" many of the fitness gains, such as better endurance, strength and ease in walking up hills, that they had enjoyed when they exercised faithfully.

STEP AWAY FROM THE TELEVISION!

A spring 2010 study found that people who watched television for more than four hours a day were 80 percent more likely to die from heart disease and atherosclerosis than those who restricted their TV watching to two hours or less per day.

One possible solution: If you must watch your programs, invest in a treadmill and walk away your TV time.

WHICH ACTIVITIES TO CHOOSE?

Your choice of exercise depends on many factors—your schedule, your weight, your current heart health, family demands and your dietary needs, among others.

One important note: A well-balanced exercise program includes aerobic activity, strength training and stretching.

You're not likely to incorporate all three facets into each workout, but try to include them every week. Many experts say stretching is the most overlooked exercise segment, and it's important to our flexibility, especially as we age. Try to work a few minutes of gentle stretching into each day.

If you enjoy walking, you should aim for 8,000 to 10,000 steps, or an average of about five miles, each day—easy to track with a good pedometer. (Most people walk an average of just 3,000 to 4,000 steps per day.) That daily goal can be a real motivation, almost a game: If I take this route, how many extra steps will I add? How many steps is it from the farthest corner of the parking lot to the door of the supermarket? Which involves the most steps—mowing the lawn, or walking to the post office?

Light exercise

Activities in this category burn about four calories per minute. They include:

- Slow walking
- Light gardening
- Casual golf
- Housework
- Yoga
- Ice skating
- Ping-Pong
- Water aerobics
- Line dancing

Moderate exercise

These activities burn about seven calories a minute and include:

- Brisk walking
- Swimming
- Moderate bicycling

- Singles tennis (which can be vigorous, but is considered "moderate" because it's a start-and-stop activity, rather than continuous movement)
- Light aerobics
- Light weight training
- Shoveling snow
- Dancing

Heavy exercise

These activities burn an average of ten calories per minute and include:

- Jogging
- "Spinning" cycling
- Racquetball
- Kickboxing
- Climbing stairs
- Cross-country skiing
- Wrestling
- Heavy weight training

EXERCISING AEROBICALLY

Literally, "aerobic" means "using oxygen." This type of exercise makes your heart beat faster and sends more blood (and oxygen) through your system. It makes your muscles, including your heart, stronger and more efficient—so that, eventually, your muscles carry you and metabolize your food with ease.

What's more, stronger muscles, a higher fitness level and lower resting heart rate mean less strain on your heart as it pumps blood throughout your body. Translation: If you have high blood pressure and you exercise aerobically, over time you will become more fit and your heart will do its job without trying so hard. Gradually, your blood pressure will go down to a healthier level.

Examples of aerobic exercise are jogging, swimming and brisk walking. It's important, while you're doing these activities, to check your heart rate so that you *are* exercising aerobically. That's true cardiovascular conditioning, and the way to do it is to keep your heart beating in a target range.

Your target range is 70 to 85 percent of your maximum-safe heart rate, which is 220 minus your age. So, to figure out your best target range, simply subtract your age from 220 and calculate the numbers representing 70 and 85 percent of it. If your heart is *not* beating at 70 percent of your maximum heart rate when you exercise, you need to work a little harder—and if it's near the 85 percent mark, you should slow down a bit.

The table below will give you an approximate guideline of target pulse ranges. Fitness experts recommend that you exercise at a rate where you can comfortably carry on a conversation; you're breathing hard but not gasping for breath, and you should be able to continue at that rate for at least twenty minutes.

TARGET HEARTBEAT RANGES

Age	Maximum Heart Rate	Target Range
30	190	133–162
35	185	130–157
40	180	126–153
45	175	122–140
50	170	119–145
55	165	115–140
60	160	112–136
65	155	109–132
70	150	105–128
75	145	102–123
80	140	98–119

If you haven't been exercising recently, start slowly—select a light activity and stop after ten minutes, three times a week. The following week, see if you feel comfortable adding minutes or stepping up the activity level.

Some people become easily bored with exercise. If you're one of them, diversify your workouts. Try walking one week, bowling another, cleaning windows one day, and dancing one day. Mix it up, even during a workout, and you won't lose interest in it.

If, on the other hand, you're the kind of person who commits more easily to a set routine, by all means stick with one or two exercises that work for you. If the only aerobic exercise that interests you is jogging, there's no point in trying to force yourself to work out on an elliptical machine. Keep doing the exercises that will keep you moving, even if it means doing the same one-exercise routine every day.

GET STRONGER WITH STRENGTH TRAINING

You may have heard the statistic: Americans lose up to 20 percent of their muscle strength by the time they reach the age of fifty, then up to 30 percent more before the age of seventy. After age forty, they lose six pounds of muscle every decade—no wonder we think our bodies have changed! It's a downward spiral, unless we take action to stop it.

Strength training can counter the muscle loss *and* help you lose excess weight. The more muscle mass you can build, the better your metabolic rate will be, and the more efficiently you will burn calories and maintain a healthy weight.

Aerobic exercise helps because it burns calories, but it's weight training that addresses your muscle strength. In a month or two of lifting free weights, you can see an enormous difference regardless of your age. Strength training is an activity you can perform in your living room, and your "free weights" can be cans of soup. You can find hundreds of videos and books outlining strength-building programs for people of all ages and physical conditions. You'll also find classes and expertise at your local YMCA, YWCA and recreation centers.

STRETCH AWAY YOUR STIFFNESS!

If you can't touch your toes easily, you're not flexible.

We're told that we lose up to 5 percent of our flexibility every decade. That means we still can walk around and move in and out of our cars, but you might catch yourself grunting at the sudden movement, because it awakens some stiff ache.

Stretching is an individual matter. We all get "stiff" in different ways. Working with a personal trainer, at least when you begin exercising, is a great experience for those who can manage it. But if you don't have the time or resources for a trainer, you can find dozens of excellent videos and books on the market. We recommend the classic, *Stretching* by Bob Anderson (Random House, 30th anniversary ed., 2010).

When you begin stretching, remember these important tips.

One, don't bounce during your stretch. Move slowly in the direction you've chosen, and try to hold the pose for thirty seconds.

And two, don't hold your breath while you stretch. We all tend to do that, but try to remember to breathe normally; it will help you stretch a bit farther and be more comfortable in the movement.

SLOW DOWN FOR SAFETY

As you get into your exercise program, TLC recommends these guidelines to keep you healthy and avoid injuries.

- Begin each exercise period with five minutes of slow movement. That could mean walking in place, some arm lifts and gentle kicks, or even a standing activity such as washing dishes. Easing into your routine in this way gives your muscles a chance to warm up.

- End each session with another five minutes of gentle moves, so your muscles can cool down.

- Be alert for body signals. Don't work through pain. Discern the difference between your "normal" aches and the pain of an injured joint or pulled muscle. If you feel pain, stop that activity for a few days until your joints and muscles recover; in most instances an over-the-counter painkiller will heal such minor problems.

- Listen to the weather forecast. You're going to work up a bit of heat as your exercise session continues; dress appropriately for hot or cold days.

- Always hydrate. Carry a small water bottle, even if you're only walking one mile. You will be amazed at how energizing a good gulp of water can be! Drink plenty of water before and after the workout, too.

- Heed any symptoms or warning signals. Especially if you've had heart problems in the past, talk with your doctor about the activity level, duration and kinds of exercise that will do you the most good. If you feel suddenly dizzy, want to faint, or feel pain or pressure in your upper body while you exercise or shortly after you've finished, call 911 immediately.

- Carry a cell phone with you when you exercise away from home.

- Exercise can be a good family activity. Before- or after-dinner walks are a great way to pursue your wellness goals and spend time together.

- Be safe. Don't walk, jog or bicycle at night.

CUT THE STRESS

It shouldn't surprise you to hear that your brain and physical responses are closely linked. We hear of someone's loss and we cry. We read a funny story and laugh out loud on the train. When someone jumps out of the bushes and shouts, "Gotcha!" our hearts race.

Financial pressures, proud moments, intellectual challenges—all of these activities involve *thinking*, but they also generate a physical response. One of our strongest responses happens when we encounter stress; our bodies produce a quick spurt of adrenaline and, over time, result in elevated inflammation (CRP) and higher cholesterol levels. The landmark INTERHEART study of 2004, in fact, found that about 30 percent of our heart attack risk is due to stress.

The good news is, the same study found that regular exercise, a sense of humor and optimism, a reliable support group and—surprise!—a relationship with a pet, all can work together to help counter that stress-related risk.

One way to start cutting stress is to work a little less. A study of about 6,000 British government workers, released in May 2010 and published in the *European Heart Journal*, found that those who worked three or more hours of overtime each day had a 60 percent increased risk of heart disease, compared to their co-workers who rarely or never worked extra hours. The study covered both white-collar and blue-collar workers; those in professional positions who regularly worked overtime exhibited "type A" behavior traits such as hostility, aggression, competitiveness, psychological distress and sleep problems.

Men in the study were six times more likely to fall in the 46 percent of subjects who regularly worked overtime, and married people of both genders were nine times more likely to be in that group.

So, does this mean you should rush to the pet store to buy a Yorkie? Probably not—but researchers concluded that taking time to read a novel, play with your children, enjoy a spa treatment and talk with friends about matters other than problems at work all can give you perspective and help bring down the stress a notch.

MEDITATION, THE GREAT COMFORTER

If you've not meditated in the past, it's difficult to comprehend the enormous impact that just a few minutes of such deliberate relaxation can have on your overall wellness. Just being still and focusing on one thought isn't easy at first—but if you can spend just a few minutes each day, totally quiet with yourself, you will see that the simplest meditation can give you a feeling of control, of being more grounded and centered, that can last the entire day.

In Chapter 6, you learned about mindful eating. Did you try it? It's an easy way to control the amount of food you eat at every meal, you remember, by focusing on every detail of every bite you take in.

Well, mindfulness meditation works the same way: You focus on one thing, usually your breath. What happened earlier this morning is part of your history, so you needn't worry about it now. What happens later today can't be known, so in mindfulness meditation you focus your awareness on what you know *here* and *now*.

It's good for your cholesterol, too: In a 2009 study published in *Stroke*, the journal of the American Heart Association, sixty African American men and women with high blood pressure either practiced meditation each morning and evening, or were in a control group. After seven months, those who meditated lowered their plaque levels and reduced their risk of having a heart attack by 11 percent and their risk of a stroke by up to 15 percent. The control group experienced no plaque reduction at all. Other published studies had similar results—participants who meditated lowered their cholesterol levels, presumably because their meditation practices reduced their stress.

Try a brief meditation now, after you finish reading this section.

1) Make yourself as comfortable as possible. Put your feet flat on the floor, rest your hands on your legs or the arms of the chair, and sit "comfortably straight" in your seat.

2) Set aside the book and shut your eyes. Breathe very slowly, counting to seven as you inhale. Hold that breath for three seconds, then exhale, again counting to seven.

3) Concentrate on your breath, the way you focused on a bite of food when you tried mindful eating. Is it warm on your lips, or cool? Is the temperature the same when you inhale, as when you're exhaling? Can you detect any aromas? What sound does your breath make?

4) Try to "breathe" through your belly button, allowing your stomach to inflate as you inhale, rather than your chest.

5) Don't try too hard not to think other thoughts. But when they do intrude, picture a gentle hand pushing them away, out of your awareness, until you're finished meditating.

6) Try to continue meditating for five minutes. Once you get the hang of it, you will get better at not permitting other thoughts and really relaxing as you meditate. (Some people find that they relax a little *too* much when they meditate. It's not supposed to be a nap session! Meditate when your energy is high and you're least likely to fall asleep. For most people that would be early in the morning.)

YOU JUST CAN'T SMOKE ANYMORE

It seems appropriate, somehow, to end with the simplest message of all: Don't smoke. It's not only your lungs that are ruined by smoking; it's actually responsible for about one-third of all deaths from heart disease! Here's what smoking does to your cardio system:

- It lowers your HDL "good" cholesterol by up to 4 mg/L in men and 6 mg/dL in women—which means an 8 percent higher risk of heart disease for men and 18 percent for women.

- Smoking encourages the formation of blood clots.

- Smoking forces carbon monoxide into the blood, lowering the amount of oxygen it carries through the body.

- Smoking damages the arterial lining, causing inflammation.

Nicotine is the toxin we know about in cigarettes, but smoke also introduces carbon monoxide, lead, arsenic, cadmium, hydrogen cyanide and at least 4,000 other poisonous chemicals into our bodies.

Secondhand smoke, too, is poisonous; it causes upwards of 40,000 deaths to nonsmokers each year because their exposure to secondhand smoke led to heart disease. Nor are cigars harmless—they contain more than twenty times more nicotine than cigarettes.

If you smoke now and want to stop, talk to your doctor about your options. Thousands of people—perhaps millions— have found success with nicotine gum, the nicotine patch, and medications. You also can find a wealth of stop-smoking information at these websites:

- www.smokefree.gov. Sponsored by the U.S. government, SmokeFree offers online and phone support, as well as resources on the site.

- www.americanheart.org. The AHA website provides information on quitting and, of course, much info on heart health.

- www.lungusa.org. Website of the American Lung Association.

- www.cancer.org. More stop-smoking information on this website of the American Cancer Society.

AFTERWORD

"You'll die of something," the doctor told me a year ago, "but it won't be heart disease. You've had the same cholesterol scores for twenty-five years."

I was a little surprised at his confidence in my heart health. I only dabble at exercise, I've never met a French fry I didn't love, and I smoked for 20-plus years. (I quit nearly 20 years ago, but . . .) Still, I've never pictured myself with heart disease. All of my aunts, uncles, and half of my immediate family died of cancer. That's the shoe I've always thought would drop.

Then, a few months ago, my younger sister, Margie, told me her LDL cholesterol was around 250, "but my other lipids are okay." Her doctor told her to start exercising. That doctor didn't know that, several years earlier, Margie had taken an "ultra-sensitive C-reactive protein" test, an inflammation measure, and her CRP level—a predictor of heart disease—was significantly high.

When I remarked that she was the first in our family to have heart problems, she said, "Well, not exactly . . ." She reminded me of Dad's heart attack during his cancer treatment back in the early 1980s, and Aunt Marie's pacemaker in the late '70s. Grandma Dakovich died in her sleep—possibly from a heart attack—before she turned 60, and Grandma Mihaly's heart gave out as she napped on her birthday. Maybe we weren't just the cancer family.

What I've found so interesting as I researched this book is the pace at which modern medicine discovers new twists in the fight against heart disease. One week, short people—those under 5-feet-3 inches—were found to have a 50 percent higher heart disease risk. Another week, researchers in Alabama found that kudzu, "the vine that's eating the South," might be useful in treating metabolic syndrome. A few weeks later, scientists at Northwestern University designed synthetic HDL, the "good" cholesterol.

I could recite a dozen examples. That's why health journalism is so exciting right now. Rapid-fire discoveries—new treatments, new medicines, new angles on old solutions—are released constantly. Last year's illness gives way to this week's findings and we move on, healthier all the time.

In the end, it's about your relationship with your own health. We all need to pay close attention to our bodies, trusting the signals, collecting information. We can't be too complacent; good health is an opportunity we don't want to miss.

If we did our jobs, *The Complete Guide to Lowering Your Cholesterol: Your All-in-One Resource for a Heart-Healthy Life* will be useful to you as you pursue glowing health! We hope this book helps you feel more empowered than ever—in taking charge of your own well-being, gathering the most reliable and up-to-date information, and, along with a health professional whom you trust, making the best decisions possible for your healthy future.

Be well, and take heart. When you have a moment, let's follow each other on Twitter; I'm @marymihaly.

RESOURCES

American Heart Association. 2002. AHA recommends fish oil supplements. *Circulation*, 106:2747–2757.

American Heart Association. 2010. Inflammation, heart disease and stroke: the role of C-reactive protein. Online: www.americanheart.org/presenter.jhtml?identifier=4648.

American Heart Association. Lyon diet heart study. Online: www.americanheart.org/presenter.jhtml?identifier=4655.

American Heart Association's Medtronic Foundation. Be The Beat, Online: www.BeTheBeat.org.

Appel, Lawrence J., et al. 2005. Effects of protein, mono-unsaturated fat, and carbohydrate intake on blood pressure and serum lipids: results of the OmniHeart randomized trial. *Journal of the American Medical Association,* 294 (19) 2455–2464.

Becker, David, M.D., et al. 2009. Red Yeast Rice for Dyslipidemia in Statin-Intolerant Patients. *Annals of Internal Medicine,* 150: 830–839.

Cancer Project, www.cancerproject.org. January 2009. The five most unhealthful Super Bowl party foods.

Clarke, Robert, et al. 2009. Life expectancy in relation to cardiovascular risk factors: 38-year follow-up of 19,000 men in the Whitehall study. *British Medical Journal*, 339:b3513. doi:10.1136/bmj.b3513.

Conkling, Winifred. 2009. *The Complete Guide to Living Well with Diabetes.* St. Martin's Paperbacks.

Devries, Stephen R., M.D. 2007. *What Your Doctor May Not Tell You about Cholesterol: The Latest Natural Treatments and Scientific Advances in One Breakthrough Program.* Warner Wellness.

Ditscheid, B. et al. 2005. Cholesterol metabolism is affected by calcium phosphate supplementation in humans. *Journal of Nutrition*, 135: 1678–1682.

Engler, Marguerite, M.D., et al. 2005. DHA improves quality of cholesterol in children. *The American Journal of Cardiology*, 95:869–871.

Flammer, Andreas J., M.D., et al. 2007. Dark chocolate improves coronary vasomotion and reduces platelet reactivity. *Circulation*, 116:2376–2382.

Go, Alan S., M.D., et al. Health plan reports major drop in heart attacks. *New England Journal of Medicine*. Online: www.nlm.nih.gov/medlineplus/news/fullstory_99782.html

Hennekens, Charles H., M.D., et al. 1998. Fish consumption and risk of sudden cardiac death. *Journal of the American Medical Association*, 279:23.

Hommel, M., et al. 1999. Alcohol for stroke prevention? *New England Journal of Medicine*, 341:1605–1606.

Howard, Barbara V., PhD., et al. 2006. Low-fat dietary pattern and risk of cardiovascular disease: the women's health initiative randomized controlled dietary modification trial. *Journal of the American Medical Association*, 295:655–666.

Jambazian, P., et al. 2005. Almonds in the diet simultaneously improve plasma alpha-tocopherol concentrations and reduce plasma lipids. *Journal of the American Dietetic Association*, 105(3):449–454.

Jenkins, D.J., et al. 2005. Direct comparison of a dietary portfolio of cholesterol-lowering foods with a statin in hypercholesterolemic participants. *American Journal of Clinical Nutrition.* 81(2):380–387.

Katz, D.L., et al. 2004. Oats, antioxidants and endothelial function in overweight, dyslipidemic adults. *Journal of the American College of Nutrition*, 23(5):397–403.

LaMarche, B., et al. 2004. Combined effects of a dietary portfolio of plant sterols, vegetable protein, viscous fibre and almonds on LDL particle size. *British Journal of Nutrition.* 92(4):657–663.

Malaguarnera, M., et al. 2009. L-Carnitine supplementation reduces oxidized LDL cholesterol in patients with diabetes. *American Journal of Clinical Nutrition.* 89 (1):71–6.

Mercken, E.M., et al. 2010. A toast to your health, one drink at a time. *American Journal of Clinical Nutrition.* 92:1–2.

Mitchell, Deborah. 2008. *A Woman's Guide to Vitamins, Herbs, and Supplements.* St. Martin's Paperbacks.

Mohaupt, M.G., et al. 2009. Association between statin-associated myopathy and skeletal muscle damage. *Canadian Medical Association Journal,* 181(1–2). doi:10.1503/cjaj.081705.

Neal, William, M.D., et al. 2010. Universal versus targeted cholesterol screening among youth: the CARDIAC project. *Pediatrics,* doi:10. 1542.peds/2009–2546.

Padilla, J., et al. The effect of acute exercise on endothelial function following a high-fat meal. 2006. *European Journal of Applied Psychology,* 98(3):256–262.

Park, Y., et al. 2009. Erythrocyte fatty acid profiles can predict acute non-fatal myocardial infarction. *British Journal of Nutrition,* 102:1355–1361.

Ridker, Paul M., et al. 2005. Non-HDL cholesterol, apolipoproteins A-I and B100, standard lipid measures, lipid ratios, and CRP as risk factors for cardiovascular disease in women. *Journal of the American Medical Association,* 294:326–333.

Rovelli, F., et al. 2002. GISSI prevention trial. *Circulation,* 105:1897–1903.

Ruano, J., et al. 2007. Intake of phenol-rich virgin olive oil improves the postprandial prothrombotic profile in hypercholesterolemic patients. *American Journal of Clinical Nutrition,* 86(2):341–346.

Sabaté, Joan, M.D., et al. 2010. Nut consumption and blood lipid levels: a pooled analysis of 25 intervention trials. *Archives of Internal Medicine,* 170(9):821–827.

Shai, Iris, R.D., Ph.D., et al. 2010. Dietary intervention to reverse carotid atherosclerosis. *Circulation,* 121:1200–1208.

Shan, B., et al. 2005. Antioxidant capacity of 26 spice extracts and characterization of their phenolic constituents. *Journal of Agricultural and Food Chemistry,* 53 (20): 7749–7759.

Siri-Tarino, Patty W., et al. 2010. Saturated fat, carbohydrate, and cardiovascular disease. *American Journal of Clinical Nutrition,* 91:502–509.

Smit, L.A., et al. 2010. Conjugated linoleic acid in adipose tissue and risk of myocardial Infarction. *American Journal of Clinical Nutrition,* 92:34–40.

Sonberg, Lynn. 2006. *Foods That Combat Heart Disease.* Avon Books.

Speizer, Frank, et al. Ongoing. Fish and omega-3 fatty acid intake and risk of coronary heart disease in women. *Journal of the American Medical Association,* 287(14): 1815

Tapsell, Linda C., et al. 2004. Including walnuts in a low-fat, modified-fat diet improves HDL cholesterol-to-total cholesterol ratios in patients with type 2 diabetes. *Diabetes Care.* Online: http://care.diabetesjournals.org/content/27/12/2777.abstract.

U.S. Department of Health and Human Services, National Institutes of Health, National Center for Complementary and Alternative Medicine. Online: Using dietary supplements wisely. Online: http://nccam.nih.gov/health/supplements/wiseuse.htm

U.S. Department of Health and Human Services, National Institutes of Health, National Heart, Lung, and Blood Institute, National Cholesterol Education Program. Online: Third report of the expert panel on detection, evaluation, and treatment of the high blood cholesterol in adults (adult treatment panel III): full report. www.nhlbi.nih.gov/guidelines/cholesterol/atp_iii.htm

U.S. Department of Health and Human Services, National

Institutes of Health, National Heart, Lung, and Blood Institute, National Cholesterol Education Program. Online: Your guide to lowering cholesterol with therapeutic lifestyle changes (TLC). www.nhlbi.nih.gov/health/public/heart/chol/chol_tlc.htm

University of Minnesota, Global Summit on Whole Grains. www.wholegrain.umn.edu.

Virtanen, Marianna, Ph.D., et al. 2010. Overtime work and incident coronary heart disease: the Whitehall II prospective cohort study. *European Heart Journal*. Online:eurheartj.oxfordjournals.org/content/early/2010/05/04/eurheartj.ehq124.

Vos, Miriam, M.D., et al. 2010. Caloric sweetener consumption and dyslipidemia among U.S. adults. *Journal of the American Medical Association*. 303:1490–1497.

Warensjö, E., et al. 2010. Biomarkers of milk fat and the risk of myocardial infarction in men and women: a prospective, matched case-control study. *American Journal of Clinical Nutrition*. 92:194–202.

Watson, R. R. 2003. Pycnogenol and cardiovascular health. Review. *Evidence Based Integrative Medicine*, 1:27–32.

Zittermann, A. 2006. Vitamin D and disease prevention with special reference to cardiovascular disease. *Progress in Biophysics and Molecular Biology*, 92(1):39–48.